ARKANA

LOVE, SEX, AND YOUR HEART

Dr. Alexander Lowen is the creator of bioenergetics, a revolutionary method of psychotherapy designed to restore the body to its natural freedom and spontaneity through a regimen of exercise. The foremost exponent of this method of incorporating direct work on the body with the psychoanalytic process, Dr. Lowen practices psychiatry in New York and Connecticut and is the executive director of the Institute of Bioenergetic Analysis. He and his wife live in New Canaan, Connecticut. Dr. Lowen's other titles include *Depression and the Body*, *Pleasure*, and *Bioenergetics*, all of which are available from Arkana.

LOVE, SEX, and YOUR HEART

Alexander Lowen, M.D.

PENGUIN

ARKANA

ARKANA
Published by the Penguin Group
Penguin Books USA Inc., 375 Hudson Street,
New York, New York 10014, U.S.A.
Penguin Books Ltd, 27 Wrights Lane,
London W8 5TZ, England
Penguin Books Australia Ltd, Ringwood, Victoria, Australia
Penguin Books Canada Ltd, 10 Alcorn Avenue,
Toronto, Ontario, Canada M4V 3B2
Penguin Books (N.Z.) Ltd, 182–190 Wairau Road,
Auckland 10, New Zealand

Penguin Books Ltd, Registered Offices:
Harmondsworth, Middlesex, England

First published in the United States of America
by Macmillan Publishing Company 1988
Published in Arkana 1994

1   3   5   7   9   10   8   6   4   2

PUBLISHER'S NOTE
The ideas, procedures, and suggestions contained in this book
are not intended as a substitute for consulting with your physician.
All matters regarding your health require medical supervision.

THE LIBRARY OF CONGRESS HAS CATALOGUED THE HARDCOVER AS FOLLOWS:
Lowen, Alexander.
Love, sex, and your heart/Alexander Lowen.
p.   cm.
Includes bibliographical references.
ISBN 0-02-575891-8 (hc.)
ISBN 0 14 01.9478 9 (pbk.)
1. Sex.   2. Love.   3. Sex (Biology).   4. Heart—Diseases.   I. Title.
HQ21.L63   1988
306.7—dc19   87–33623

Printed in the United States of America
Set in Sabon

CONTENTS

We all recognize the heart as a symbol of love. But is the relationship between the heart and love only symbolic? Or is there a real and vital connection?

Most people have experienced not only a rapid heartbeat in the presence of a loved one but also the heaviness of heart that follows a lovers' quarrel. Moreover, it is common practice in all cultures to place a hand over the heart when talking about love, as if to locate the physical sensations that accompany the emotion. If the heart is involved in every experience of love, as it seems to be, then we must assume that such expressions as a "heart filled with love" also describe a physical phenomenon.

What validity can one then give to the concept of heartbreak? Although hearts do not fall to pieces when love is rejected or a loved one is lost, clearly something breaks in such situations. Is there such a thing as a closed heart or an open heart? These questions are important to an understanding not only of our feelings but also for the health of the heart. Assuming that the connection between the heart and love is real, as I do throughout this book, it can be hypothesized that a heart without love must inevitably languish and die. My belief in this conviction stems from my experience as a doctor helping patients in their struggle to open their hearts to love and to find some joy in life. Some of their case histories will be presented in this study.

What about sex? If we contend, as some people do, that love and sex are two separate functions, then we must assume that the heart is no more involved in the sex act than it is in any other physical activity. In this view, the heart's function of pumping the blood through the body to provide the tissues with oxygen and nutrients and to remove waste products must be seen as purely mechanical. Here again, however, we run up against the common language, which speaks of sex as lovemaking, implying a direct connection between love and sex and, by extension, between the heart and the genital organs.

It is the purpose of this book to elucidate these connections so that the reader may see how his emotional life is tied to his physical being and how his physical health is dependent on his emotional well-being. It is my hope that understanding the causes of the fear of love will help the reader become a more loving person, thus ensuring the health of his heart. Without such knowledge, all our efforts to ensure the health of our hearts fail to go to the core of the problem.

We shall therefore start by examining the nexus between the heart and love, a relationship that has been recognized and expressed over the centuries by poets, philosophers, and religious teachers.

As a clinical cardiologist I have seen and worked with many cases of heart disease. Over the years it became apparent to me that coronary heart disease in general is a silent, ubiquitous disease. Symptoms are usually a late manifestation, and sudden cardiac death is frequently the first symptom of coronary insufficiency. This obviously presents a dilemma for the practicing cardiologist. The preventive aspects of dealing with such a devastating illness recently have become the focus of contemporary cardiology. One's predetermined risk and habit profiles have become important variables in the relationship between life-style and cardiovascular disease. But despite all the studies linking smoking, high levels of blood cholesterol, hypertension, and adult diabetes to coronary artherosclerosis, I was convinced that these risk factors, although highly significant, really did not completely explain the nature of this illness.

Over the years, and especially within the last decade, a considerable amount of research has been undertaken in an effort to discover the causes of atherosclerotic cardiovascular disease—a unique phenomenon of twentieth-century people. This research has been mostly of a statistical nature, demonstrating a connection between risk factor profiles and subsequent cardiac disease. Additional research studies, however, have disclosed that certain individuals are more prone to coronary heart disease than others. Such disease-prone individuals have a special pattern of behavior and unusual susceptibility to emotional stress. Emotional stress seemed to me to be the most important determinate of cardiac illness, so when Friedman and Rosenman published their findings about Type A coronary-prone behavior and its predisposition to coronary artery disease, it confirmed my belief in the dominant role of stress and behavior in heart disease.

Cardiologists are particularly prone to heart disease because of the stressful nature of their work. As a clinical cardiologist I became aware of patterns of destructive behavior in my patients that labeled individuals "prone to developing coronary heart disease." What I didn't expect to discover, however, was that I was wearing that label myself. This awareness was horrifying. I knew that I had been competitive, an achiever, and a hard worker. I also recognized myself as a Type A individual. As a man in my late thirties, aggressive and successful, I suddenly realized that my own mortality was being revealed to me through my patients.

Traditional cardiovascular risk factors frequently were not found in victims of coronary heart disease. Typically, it was one's behavior that became the catalyst of the disease process. Emotional factors operating on a physiological level affected the process of heart disease. It is well known that mind and body influence each other. What one thinks can elicit an emotional response to which the body responds. Thus, personality issues are key elements found in almost every illness. Unventilated emotion or affect, for instance, eventually damages the body and its physiological system. In high blood pressure, the major repressed emotions are anger, hostility, and rage. Some coronary-prone individuals, in addition to repressing anger and hostility, have also struggled with the heartbreaking experience of the loss of love and subsequent loss of a vital connection. Such feelings of heartbreak imply great sorrow, grief, and anguish, which are subsequently expressed in one's evolving behavior, character, and body. Thus, it became clear to me that heart disease is a process that doesn't just happen. Rather, it is frequently influenced by emotional issues, conscious and unconscious conflicts. Therefore, such behavioral analysis became the focus of my interest and energies. I was also able to view it as a challenge to find the causative factor one might identify and modify in order to enhance and prolong the lives of my patients as well as my own. Also, this realization that I was setting myself up for coronary illness made me decide to enter therapy, with a view to investigating and changing these negative aspects of my behavior.

My search sent me back to my childhood, and a recognizable pattern developed. I was the third of four children. When I was four years old, my sister was born, and around that time I started a course of multiple childhood illnesses and accidents. Were those incidents a maladaptive way to achieve contact and love from a mother who must have had her hands full with a new baby and a growing family? Through the years I can still feel that yearning for my mother's attention aad soothing. Her "unavailability" to me resulted in the experience of my first heartbreak. The traumatic sadness that followed was repressed, but somehow my body remembered the truth. The soft vulnerability of the child evolved into the rigidity of a heavily armored chest, as if to protect my heart. I know my mother loved me dearly, but at that young age I was unable to understand her needs and focused only on my own. I sought her approval and love and hoped that by being "a good boy, a good student, an athlete, and an achiever," I would gain them. *Success* would bring me love, I thought. I developed a false connection between the two that carried through to adulthood. This connection influenced the process of Type A behavior that ultimately could result in my demise.

After medical school I went through an internship in psychiatry and medicine, two years of residency in medicine, and two years of specialized training in cardiology. I became a highly trained technical invasive cardiologist and felt extremely confident in what I was doing. I became a workaholic. The passion in my life was my job, for it had given me a place in the universe.

Over a short period of time, however, in the midst of this success, I felt myself burning out. I was in an internal struggle to achieve and perform at the expense of my feelings. Although I didn't recognize it, I was a driven man. I denied my fatigue and my pain, something I had done in my adolescence to prove myself a good student and athlete. In this pursuit of success and achievement, was I really seeking approval and love? Was I trying to prove myself worthy of love? I had carried this need through the years and saw it again and again in many of my patients. Many chased this need to heart disease and death.

The challenge I now gave myself was to alter the self-destructive Type A coronary behavior pattern. Actually, the awareness and recognition that I possessed this behavior was enlightening, for it was this awareness that gave me the strength to find a curative alternative.

In the mid-seventies, I was fortunate to hear lectures and seminars given by my colleagues on behavior and cardiovascular disease. One lecturer, Robert Elliot, a cardiologist and author of the book *Is It Worth Dying For?* had a tremendous impact on me. After these encounters I pursued many self-awareness seminars. In 1978, for instance, I attended an international symposium in London, England, on stress and tension. It was extremely provocative and opened me up to some of the nontraditional approaches toward healing. The West Germans, for example, were integrating biofeedback with their treatments; the Swedes were utilizing massage, the Swiss introduced Lamaze, the Asians focused on meditation, while the Americans were teaching progressive relaxation. I was able to see each of these methods as a positive way of assuaging emotion and calming the nervous system. They all had merit.

Over the next few years I was fortunate to conduct stress-and-illness workshops with an internist, Dr. Brendan Montano, and a psychotherapist, Holly Hatch. These group interactions, utilizing Gestalt therapeutic technique, were helpful in teaching susceptible individuals how to cope with life. Group awareness training had a tremendous impact on healing, particularly when individuals "saw themselves" in other people. After being involved in several workshops, I began to publish some of my own data in the medical literature. My patients became my best teachers. During this time I realized I needed to pursue specialized training in the field of psychotherapy. The more I investigated the connection between mind, emotion, and heart, the more uneasy and inadequate I became. The subject was simply vast, unexplored, and uncharted.

I spent two years in Gestalt therapy, which helped me understand some of the background causes of my attitudes and further convinced me about the power of emotions in health and illness. In the course of this therapy I discovered the work of Alexander Lowen. Bioenergetic analysis, which he founded, is a body-oriented analytic therapy that focuses upon muscular tensions in the body that are the physical counterpart of the emotional conflicts in the personality. Just as one can tell the age of a tree by counting the internal rings on the stump, a bioenergetic therapist, like Lowen, can determine the history of a person by looking at the body. In bioenergetic analysis, the therapist can determine where tension is located and where energy is blocked. This blockage keeps people from experiencing their full potential of aliveness. By utilizing various techniques and exercises to charge and discharge the body, the bioenergetic therapist can release trapped energy, which allows for the dissipation of tension. This concept of energy and its application to individuals prone to heart disease were so intriguing and exciting, that I decided to undergo therapy with Dr. Lowen. Through his teachings it soon became apparent to me that my body was quite tense, that I was not breathing deeply, and that I was not fully experiencing or expressing my own feelings.

My therapy with Dr. Lowen focused on the rigidity of my body. Although during the first few months my body was resistant and under the control of my head, Lowen worked on my breathing, which induced feeling. He placed me over a bioenergetic stool and had me use my voice in such a way as to assuage the energy in my chest. This had a positive effect in reducing the stress and tension in my thoracic cage. He then began to focus on my diaphragm, jaw, and pelvis. Several months of such body work uncovered suppressed emotion and muscular tension. Gradually a softening in my body occurred. Crying released tension, inducing an expansive quality in my chest. Over the subsequent years I found my heart opening. I guess the feminine side of my character was evolving. The growth was tremendous. The pain of therapy eventually led to the discovery of pleasure. I began to experience more feeling. My emotional and physical well-being heightened, and my body seemed to come alive. I began to experience my real self. This journey of self-discovery was exhilarating.

With these new insights I began to look at my cardiac patients from the point of view of what went on in their chests, how much tension was located in their bodies, how well they breathed, what their early life experiences were with relation to loss of love, and what their current experiences were with love. My work now evolved on a different level. I began to work with my patients on a body level utilizing the knowledge that I had gained from Lowen. Bioenergetic analysis became a tremendous tool in the total assessment of each person and his illness. Although I continued to take a history from a patient, I now began to focus on his breathing, eye contact, the quality of the patient's energy, the feeling in his handshake, the movement of his diaphragm, his tone of voice, and signs of held-in emotion in his body. Analysis of the jaw structure, for instance, gave me clues to the level of the patient's held-in anger. The look in his eyes gave me information concerning sadness and fear. Thus, by looking at body structures, I became more aware of patients' issues and illnesses. I was becoming a more effective physician and healer. With such new insights, Dr. Lowen and I founded the New England Heart Center to arrive at a bioenergetic understanding of cardiac illness and the individuals who are prone to it.

My experience with Dr. Lowen has become an exciting chapter in my life. His teachings have opened up innovative, creative dimensions in the treatment of heart disease. At age seventy-six, he is a living testimony of his work. During the summer of 1987 he took me sailing on Long Island Sound, and we discussed our research. As he hoisted the sails and navigated the boat, I viewed a vibrant, energetic man who was fluid, soft, and yielding. As I experienced the wind and the spray upon my face, Lowen talked about living and feeling. As the boat glided over the waves, I had the feeling that I was participating in a sailing experience with a master. Just as a sailor navigates with masterly skill, a psychotherapist like Lowen frequently navigates through the "uncharted waters" of a patient's memories that had long since been forgotten. As I watched Lowen sail his boat, I experienced a tranquillity. . . . I will always be indebted to him for that day.

STEPHEN SINATRA, M.D.

PART ONE

The Fulfillment of Love

There is probably no concept in the English language that is used in as many different ways as *love*. Some use it to denote a general surrender of the self. Others use it in a very selfish way, to express their need to be accepted and cared for or to possess and control another person.

Love can be considered an attitude or an action, but we must recognize it as a *feeling*—and therefore a physiological process in the body. To understand love, we need to understand this physiological process. As in any physiological process, its aim is to further the well-being of the organism, which is experienced as pleasure and joy. The fulfillment of love is the joy that is felt most intensely when two people who love each other come together.

In Part 1 we will examine how love is fulfilled and how it is frustrated.

CHAPTER 1

Love Is at the Heart of Life

Since earliest times, the heart has been a powerful symbol in man's thinking. The Latin word for heart, *cor,* is the basis for the English word *core,* which is defined as the central part of an object. The interchangeability of the words heart and core is apparent in such common expressions as "to get to the heart of the matter." Most people regard the heart as the core of their being, similar to the hub of a wheel. Thus, when a person is said to have had a "change of heart," we assume that his whole attitude has undergone a transformation.

The heart symbolizes not only humanity's emotional center but also its spiritual center. The heart is believed by many to be the source of life. A Jewish mystic said, "Know thou that the heart is the source of life, and is placed in the center of the body as the Holy of Holies."[1] Since God is also believed to be the source of life, it must follow that God resides in the heart. Thus, Upanishadic teaching advises, "Enter the lotus of the heart and meditate there on the presence of the Brahman."[2]

3

According to George S. J. Mahoney, a Christian theologian, "the heart in scriptural language is the seat of human life, of all that teaches us in the depths of our personality. . . . It is in our heart that we meet God in an I-Thou relationship."[3] Brother David Steindl Rast concurs: "When we really find our heart, we find the realm where we are intimately one with self, with others and also with God."[4] The Upanishad also locates the self in the heart, at the very core of spirituality: "Verily the Self is the heart. . . . He who knows this goes in the celestial realm every day."[5] Metaphorical, spiritual, and philosophical as these teachings may be, there must be some actual physical basis for this repeated connection between the human heart and the source of life. That basis would appear to be the heartbeat itself, the rhythmic pulse that conveys life-giving blood through the body. It is the clearest manifestation of the life force in the human organism. This rhythmic pulsation characterizes all living things as well as the physical universe—both sound and light, after all, travel in waves.

Although the association of the heart with love is widely recognized in our culture, cardiologists and most lay people regard that association as symbolic. A songwriter may sing, "You stole my heart," or, "I lost my heart to you," but who believes that a person can actually lose his heart or wake up to find it stolen? Yet if we think of such expressions in functional terms, they make sense. Someone "loses" his heart when he becomes so involved with another person that it no longer seems to belong to him. Every time he thinks of his loved one, he feels a sensation of joy or sadness so intimately tied to the other that it is as if the other had taken possession of his heart.

However we describe them, feelings are not flights of the imagination. They refer to actual processes in the body, which give rise to them. When we feel heavyhearted or lighthearted, coldhearted or warmhearted, something happens on a physical level in the body to make us feel that way. What happens can best be described as a decrease or increase in the body's state of excitement. Excitement makes us feel light; in its absence, we feel heavy and depressed. When the excitement relates to love, we feel it most directly in the area of the heart. The sight or thought of a loved one can make the heart feel lighter and beat faster. It can even cause the heart to skip a beat.

As long as there is life, every cell, whether of a single-cell organism or of a complex, highly structured organism like man, exists in a state of excitation. It may wax or wane, but it is always present to some degree. Such a state is most intense in the very young and least intense in the very old, which is to say that the fire of life slowly dies out as we get older. A child can become so excited that he literally jumps for joy. The same reaction is rarer in an older person, whose body has become more rigid and stiff. In death, the body's potential for excitation is extinguished.

A person's state of excitement is always visible in his body. With a high degree of excitement, more blood flows to the surface of the body, the eyes shine, skin tone improves, movements are more spontaneous, hands are warmer, the brain is activated, and the heart beats faster. In death, the eyes become dull and glazed, the body ceases to move, and the skin turns white and cold.

States of negative excitement do not evince these same effects. When the body exhibits increased activity in a state of panic, the movements are wild and uncoordinated, and the excitement is largely concentrated in the musculature and in the heart, which may race. If the fear is great enough, the person may die as the muscular system becomes paralyzed and the heart stops beating. Intense pain, which causes the body to twist and writhe, is another state of negative excitement. So is rage, which, unlike anger, has a negative effect on the body. In anger, the body is hot, and the eyes may flash with fire; in rage, the body is cold, and the eyes are black.

Positive excitement occurs during a pleasureful situation. The body is in a state of expansion, and the charge or excitation is strong at the surface of the body. Negative excitement arises in situations of fear and danger. The body is in a state of contraction, and the charge ebbs away from the surface. Respiration also differs in the two states. During pleasure, breathing is deep, easy, and relatively slow. It never becomes labored, since labored breathing is a sign of distress. However, when a person is frightened or in pain, the breathing is shallow, forced, and rapid.

The emotion of love produces the most salutary effect on the body. A person in love seems to radiate joy. The light in his eyes and the glow of his skin are due not only to the strong flow of blood to the surface of the body but also to a wave of excitation that flows to the surface, energizing the tissues.

The radiance and glow of a person in love is not a metaphorical concept, since it can be observed. Its cause is a more highly excited and more intensely pulsating state of the organs and tissues. The property of pulsation is not limited to the heart muscle. Although it is visibly manifested in breathing and less so in the peristaltic waves of the digestive tract, it occurs in all living cells and organs. Though each tissue or organ system has its own rhythm, it is coordinated with and dependent upon the basic pulsation of the heart. It is the beat of the heart that gives life to the whole body. When we feel lighthearted, all organs function better; when we feel heavyhearted, all organ systems are depressed.

In pleasure, as we have seen, the blood flows to the surface of the body, whereas in pain it flows toward the center. In situations of panic or fear, a person may respond by acting to remove the threat or danger by mobilizing the voluntary muscular system, which lies close to the skin. These muscles will then become suffused and charged with blood in preparation for action. Whether the person experiences this response as anger or as fear depends upon whether the response is a movement toward the world with the aim of restoring harmony and pleasure or one of flight away from danger.

Figure 1. The organismic response to the environment—reaching out with pleasure or withdrawing in pain

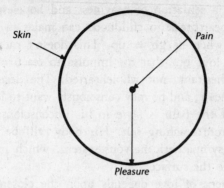

Skin

Pain

Pleasure

Pain or fear produces contraction, creating a decreased charge at the surface.
Pleasure produces expansion, creating an increased charge at the surface: skin, eyes, erogenous zones.

The movement of blood and body fluids toward or away from the surface of the body (see fig. 1) represents a person's reaction to his environment. If the environment is accepting, positive, and life affirming, the blood will rush to the surface and the person himself will reach out to make contact. In turn, these movements will engender feelings of affection and pleasure or, if the excitement is more intense, love and joy. Affection and pleasure cannot be separated from each other. We love what is pleasurable. However, love does not always produce pleasure; far too often, it results in pain. Love impels us to draw closer to the one we love, but if he or she rejects or leaves us, our pleasure quickly turns to pain. The intensity of the pain is in direct proportion to the intensity of the love. When the wholehearted love of a child for a parent meets with rejection, the pain can only be described as heartbreak.

Like all pain, heartbreak causes a withdrawal of blood from the surface of the body to the center, overloading the heart and producing a sensation of heaviness and hopelessness. The experience of heartbreak in childhood can make an individual afraid to love when he grows up. This doesn't mean that he can't or won't love but that his impulse to reach out will be tentative and hesitant, not wholehearted. The desire to love may be in his heart, and he may consciously want to love, but if the memory of the pain is alive in his unconscious, fear will prevent him from reaching out. His body will be under the control of the sympathetic nervous system, which inhibits the flow of blood to the surface.

The excitement of love depends upon the closeness of the lovers. Like the law of gravity, which states that the attraction between two bodies is inversely proportional to the square of the distance between them, the closer one gets to the beloved, the greater the excitement. The excitement is greatest when there is loving contact between two individuals.

Every pleasurable contact between two bodies leads to feelings of love. The commonplace embrace of two friends when they meet is an expression of affection that serves to cement the relationship between them. The handshake is the most informal physical contact to express a degree of positive feeling. Withholding a handshake when meeting or leaving can be regarded as an expression of coldness or hostility. Similarly, when parents withhold physical affection from their children, it cannot help but cut to the quick. Many of my patients have complained that their parents rarely touched, held, or kissed them despite the fact that they told them they were loved. Their parents may well have loved them, but the feeling was rarely expressed in a way that made my patients *feel* loved.

There are many ways to make loving contact without touching a person's body. Sound, for example, is a physical force that impinges on the body. Children are warmed and soothed by a mother's lullaby, which they perceive as an expression of love.

Spoken words of love can have the same effect, not because of the words themselves but because of the tone in which they are uttered. A warm voice expresses love as surely as a cold, harsh voice expresses hostility. The eyes are another important means of communication. We can look at people with warmth and affection or coldness and hostility. By saying that looks can kill, we recognize their power. By the same token, a fond look can touch our hearts.

For a sound to be emotionally effective, it must be heard; for a look to be effective, it must be seen. Eye contact is not a mechanical phenomenon with foreseeable results. Two people can look at each other and make no contact because nothing passes between them. When their eyes light up, however, they send out a beam that can reach across space to the other's eyes, resulting in real contact. Many of us have experienced such eye contact and know how exciting it is. Occasionally it results in what is called love at first sight. I can clearly remember that I fell in love with my wife the night I saw stars shine in her eyes. Her look touched my heart and captured me. Love impels closeness. Contact may start with a look, but if it follows a natural course, it will end in an embrace or in more intimate contact between two individuals.

Normally, areas of the body where the blood comes very close to the surface are where intimate contact is made. These are known as the erogenous zones; namely, the lips, the nipples, and the genital organs. The red color of the lips reflects the richness of their blood supply, which lies just under a thin layer of mucous membrane. When two lips meet in a kiss, the blood of each person is separated only by that thin membrane, which produces a high degree of excitement. Actually, the whole mouth, including the tongue, can be considered an erogenous zone, since the whole area is richly vascularized. Any contact with or stimulation of an erogenous area is exciting when the person is in the mood. When erogenous zones come in contact, as happens during sex, the excitement can rise to great heights.

Figure 2. The flow of blood (eros) from the heart (love) to the erogenous zones (pleasure)

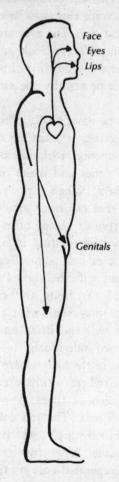

Face
Eyes
Lips

Genitals

Genital love between a man and woman should therefore be the most exciting activity of all because these organs allow the closest contact between two individuals. A similar closeness of contact occurs during the act of nursing, when the baby's mouth and mother's breast form a near-perfect union.

Figure 2 illustrates the flow of blood from the heart both upward (via the ascending aorta) and downward (via the descending aorta). In pleasure, this blood strongly suffuses the surface of the body and in erotic pleasure, it strongly excites the erogenous zones.[6] For this reason, the blood is regarded as the carrier of Eros. (For a further discussion of the blood as the carrier of Eros, see my book *The Language of the Body* [New York: Macmillan, 1971]).

Love is not limited to the sexual love between a man and woman. Love exists wherever there is pleasure and the desire for closeness. A child who loves his teddy bear will hug it to his body as if it were a living being because of the pleasure and good feeling he derives from the contact. In a similar way, we love our friends because of the pleasure and excitement we feel in their company. The love a person feels for a pet follows the same principle: The desire for closeness and contact is connected to a feeling of excitement and pleasure in that contact. To love is to feel connected, not just in an abstract way, as in the love of one's fellow man, but in a physical way, through closeness and contact.

As we noted, the most intense excitement and the greatest pleasure are possible from the genital contact between a man and woman. Such excitement and pleasure depend on these organs becoming tumescent or charged with blood, and it is the proximity of the blood to the surface that accounts for the heat of sexual passion. In the absence of engorgement, the genitals, like the skin of any other part of the body, are relatively cold. But when they are stimulated, they pulse rhythmically in response to the beating of the heart. By this reasoning, the heart is the source of Eros—or, one might also say, the home of Eros.

One of the seeming mysteries of life is the phenomenon known as love at first sight. There is no question that it occurs; too many people have reported the experience. Sometimes, however, it may be a later "sight" that turns the trick; two people who may have known each other for some time exchange a look or experience some contact that ignites the feeling of love. The only sensible explanation for this phenomenon is that each person's heart was touched and excited by a look or a kiss, sending a surge of excitement and warmth through the whole body. This feeling (call it love), like any other, impels us to action. It arouses the desire to be as close as possible to the beloved. Physical contact increases the excitement but also provides for some discharge of the tension created by the desire. Of course, a maximum discharge occurs through sexual contact, but a hug or a kiss can also act as a release.

Great pleasure does not always follow the union of lovers in a sexual embrace. Too many couples start with intense feelings of love and end with disappointment and frustration. It is much easier for most individuals to become excited than it is for them to transform that excitement into the pleasure and satisfaction that result from the full discharge of that excitement. There exists in many people an unconscious taboo against any sexual contact with a loved person. This taboo stems from childhood experiences in the Oedipal period. Its effect is to split the unity of the personality separating the feeling of love in the heart from the feeling of sexual desire in the genital apparatus. While this split is never total, it does block the fulfillment of love. We must recognize a distinction between the excitement of love and the fulfillment of love. Some unfortunate people, however, have never experienced the ecstatic excitement of falling in love that occurs when one's heart opens suddenly and fully to another person. Their hearts are closed and so cannot be reached by another person. But no heart is ever totally closed to love. Like Sleeping Beauty it may lie imprisoned by a seemingly impenetrable wall of thorns, but some prince or princess can puncture the wall and awaken the sleeping heart. When it happens, it is like a miracle.

How can one person evoke such a powerful response in another? By awakening in the unconscious a remembered feeling of pleasure and excitement. Being in love can be paradise if one's love is accepted, or it can be hell if one's love is rejected. I believe we have all known paradise and lost it. Falling in love occurs when we think we have found it again. That paradise, where all our needs were met, where there was no need to struggle or strain, was the womb. For many of us, that state of paradise continues for a short time after birth, when our mothers, like the good earth, provide for and shelter us. To some degree or other, every baby has experienced the excitement of loving contact with his mother and her body. Every baby loves his mother with all his heart and responds excitedly and pleasurably when she makes loving contact with him. That state of bliss is shattered sooner or later, but our hearts retain a longing for it.

Children have two love objects, mother and father. In the love of each, they know the joy that is possible when one loves and is loved. However, the joy of infancy and childhood doesn't last. For children who have been abused by their parents, which is not uncommon in our culture, the bliss of innocence is rudely shattered. However, if the reality of love is lost or destroyed, the dream is retained, for without it life would be bleak and empty. It is the hope of paradise regained that gives meaning to our lives. If someone comes along who resembles in some significant way the lost loved one of our childhood, the miracle seems to happen; the dream seems to become reality. In most cases, the bubble bursts. What seemed to be reality turns out to be an illusion. Why this cruel deception? What is wrong?

One of the problems encountered in any discussion of love is that the word describes two different feelings, both originating in the heart. One is the longing for closeness that stems from need. The other is the desire for closeness that stems from a fullness of heart. The feeling of love in the first case, though genuine, is infantile or childlike. It has a desperate quality because its aim is to bind the other person. Once the attachment is made, the dependent person cannot let go. But this inability to let go also expresses itself in the sexual relationship, so that there is little fulfillment in the relationship. In contrast, the love that stems from a fullness of being is mature. It doesn't bind the beloved but rather leaves him or her free.

It is not uncommon to be confused about love because of the moral injunctions we learn as children about loving our parents or loving our neighbors. In therapy, a patient may say, "I love my mother," even when his or her history contains episodes of mistreatment. After considerable analytic work, it generally turns out that the patient is angry about the mistreatment and harbors feelings of hatred for the mother. The anger and hatred have been suppressed out of guilt. Still, the recognition and acceptance of the feeling of hatred for the mother does not dispel all feelings of love. Some love persists in the heart, since mother was the giver of life and the original source of good feeling.

It is safe to conjecture that the intensity or fullness of a person's love must be reflected in the quality of the heart muscle, especially if we give credence to such expressions as warmhearted, coldhearted, softhearted, and hardhearted. The heart is a muscle like any muscle; whether it is soft or hard depends on its state of relaxation. At the same time, muscle tissue tends to lose its softness with age, which is a hardening process. A soft muscle may not be as strong as a larger, harder one in terms of its ability to work—that is, to move a weight— but it functions better because it has greater mobility and contractile power and its response is quicker and more complete. One would never say that a baby responds in a half-hearted way. A young, soft heart, capable of greater excitement, experiences a more intense feeling of love than an older heart or one that has become cold and hard.

But how does a heart become cold and hard? The answer to that question lies in the close relationship between love and hate. Hate can be described as love turned cold. [7] The process is not quick; for love to freeze, it requires repeated disappointments.

To understand this process, we must start with the impulse

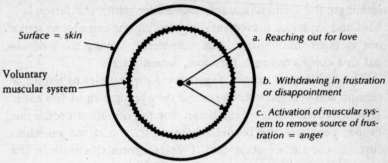

Figure 3. The reaction of anger to the frustration of the loving impulse

Surface = skin

Voluntary muscular system

a. Reaching out for love

b. Withdrawing in frustration or disappointment

c. Activation of muscular system to remove source of frustration = anger

that is at the heart of life—to reach out. If such a gesture is met with a negative response, the reaction is to become angry. In anger, the blood suffuses the musculature, as love suffuses the skin. We can illustrate this dynamic in figure 3.

If the expression of anger is successful in restoring a state of loving contact, the excitation in the muscular system is discharged. The muscles then return to a state of relaxation and softness that allows the impulse of love to reach the surface of the body again. However, when the expression of anger meets with a hostile reaction, a person has no recourse but to withdraw from the relationship, for such a response is a denial of his right to strive for the satisfaction of his needs.

This is not to say that we are obligated to accede to every expression of another's anger; but if a relationship is truly loving, we cannot deny the object of our love the right to become angry. Unfortunately, parents often deny a child that right because they construe his expressions of anger as a challenge to their authority. However, to introduce power or authority into a love relationship is to betray it. A child, because he is dependent, cannot withdraw from such a relationship. So he remains inside it, but his love turns eventually to hate; that is, the impulse to reach out is frozen like a stream in winter. In this connection we must recognize that the same muscles are involved in reaching out with the arms as in striking out, although the former is a soft movement while the latter is a hard and explosive movement. Suppressing the impulse to strike out in anger immobilizes both movements, leaving the individual in a contracted and, therefore, frozen state.

The inability to express anger leaves the muscles in a state of tension and contraction. Over time they become rigid and hard. Love may still reside in the heart, but the impulse to reach out cannot penetrate the barrier of the tight, contracted musculature, so the surface stays cold. (We recognize this state in the observation "cold hands, warm heart.") If the barrier were absolute, one might well die, for it is impossible to live without some love. Even the most hateful of the Nazis had some positive contact with other Nazis and felt some love for Hitler. But aside from such limited expressions of love, they had much hate. The dynamic that lies behind hate is shown in figure 4.

The individual is not conscious of this dynamic, nor is he aware that the hate he feels is connected to a betrayal of love he once felt. Likewise, he does not understand that some of that love, diminished though it may be, is still alive in his heart. The hate can be removed and the love reactivated by mobilizing

Figure 4. The block to loving. The impulse from the heart to love is blocked by tense and contracted surface musculature, preventing the impulse from reaching the surface.

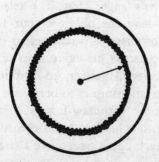

the anger locked in the tense muscles of the body. Tension in the muscles of the arms and upper back holds in anger that would be expressed through hitting and striking. Tension in the jaw muscles holds in anger that would be expressed in biting, an impulse that many babies and children feel in response to a frustrating parent. The legs are another place where anger may reside—anger that might have been discharged by kicking against a parent who handled the child's lower body callously in cleaning or in toilet training.

One other aspect of this problem deserves explanation. In figure 5, the impulse to love may be strong enough to penetrate the tense, hard muscular system, but it is torn in the process and surfaces as sadism.[8] In sadism, one hurts the beloved not in anger but as an expression of love. Many survivors of Nazi cruelty described to Wilhelm Reich a look on the faces of their tormentors that could only be described as an appeal for love and understanding. It was as if these sadists were themselves tormented people who tried to release their torment by torturing others. This look was even more distressing to the survivors than the treatment they received.

With this analysis of the vicissitudes of love, we are in a position to understand the following case, which illustrates the stresses and confusions that can arise in a marriage that seems, to all outward appearances, stable and secure.

Figure 5. The transmutation of hate to sadism

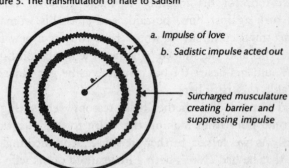

a. *Impulse of love*

b. *Sadistic impulse acted out*

Surcharged musculature creating barrier and suppressing impulse

A man in his mid-fifties named John came for a consultation because he was in a state of emotional distress. Over the past thirty years, his sexual relationship with his wife had steadily deteriorated. Although they shared a bed, they engaged in intercourse at most about once a month. Over the thirty-five years of his marriage, John had worked hard to build a successful business, and at this point he was financially independent. He and his wife had many friends, and on some level they enjoyed each other. He would have been content, he said, to continue their relationship as it was, although he admitted that such a life held no excitement for him. Fate, however, intervened in the form of a younger woman, with whom he had become involved and who had transformed his life.

Just being with this other woman, he reported, excited him. He enjoyed talking to her on the telephone and looked forward to seeing her. Normally, he said, he had trouble engaging in small talk with his acquaintances at social gatherings, but when he was with his friend, he could talk about anything or nothing for hours. Was he in love with her? He didn't know, but he thought so. And he believed she loved him, too. Of course, his sexual feelings came very much alive with her, more so than they ever had with his wife.

He came to see me because he felt torn. He would have liked to leave his wife and marry his lover, but he claimed also to love his wife and to be afraid of hurting her. He advanced other reasons, too, for his inability to make a move: His friends would turn against him, he said, and since his woman friend had two small children, he would have to raise a new family at his age; he also questioned whether their relationship would last. Would his desire for her continue as he got older? Would he be able to satisfy her?

I had some doubt whether these reasons were strong enough to prevent John from making the move toward the woman he wanted. As we talked further in subsequent meetings, he revealed that he had always been a little afraid of his wife and that she had dominated their relationship. One of the factors that had contributed to the decline of their relationship was his wife's tendency to humiliate him in public. His mother had also been the dominant figure in his childhood home and he admitted that he had been afraid of her. He couldn't hurt these women, he said, and he felt guilty if he caused them any pain. He also admitted, however, that on some level his wife looked down on him, quite unlike his lover. Still, he couldn't make the move; on the other hand, he couldn't give up his new love.

Which of the two women did he love, or did he really love them both? I had little doubt that what he felt in his new relationship was love. His heart beat faster at the thought or the sight of the woman who had awakened his sexual passion. If love is the desire to be close to another person, this was it. His wife evoked no such reaction in him, and yet it was entirely believable that he harbored some feelings in his heart for her. However, if and when he told her he loved her, I doubt that it carried much conviction, although I am sure that when he said the same words to his lover, they rang true with the vibrancy of deep feeling. How can we, then, explain the fact that by claiming to love his wife, he did not lie? If we are to understand the causes of heart disease, we need to understand the complex emotions in the human heart.

Psychiatrists use the term *ambivalent* to describe a person who experiences two opposing feelings at the same time. John was ambivalent concerning his wife. He wanted to leave her and at the same time wanted to stay with her. The effect of such ambivalence is to paralyze action. It is impossible to move if one is pulled in opposite directions at the same time. If the ambivalence persists, it creates tremendous emotional stress, which is dangerous to the heart.

How is it possible to get trapped in a love-hate relationship? When a love relationship turns sour, as it sometimes does, the healthy reaction is to end it and leave. This reaction is blocked, however, when guilt takes over. John felt guilty about leaving his wife for another woman. The notion that he might hurt her loomed large and conflicted with his image of what he ought to do. It was easier for him to dismiss the idea that he might reach out for the love of another woman than it was to accept the idea that he was angry with his wife: for dominating him, humiliating him, and showing him precious little interest in bed. By suppressing his anger, he paved the way for his love to turn into hate. But since he could no more admit he hated his wife than he could admit he was angry with her, his guilt intensified. In general, guilt stems from the suppression of feelings the superego judges to be wrong. It underlies all ambivalent attitudes and prevents the resolution of the conflict.

Psychiatrists deal with the feeling of guilt all the time in every patient. Every state of tension in the body is associated with some sense of guilt. In the absence of guilt, we would all feel worthy of love regardless of the fact that our behavior might not always meet with acceptance. We would be able to say, "I am who I am, and I accept myself." Guilt is a judgment we make that something is wrong with us, that we are not worthy of love unless we earn it by good deeds. That we feel angry toward those who have hurt us and hate those who have betrayed our love does not make us wrong. Since such reactions are biologically natural, they must be regarded as morally just. However, children, who are dependent on their parents and elders, can be easily brainwashed to believe otherwise. If a child feels unloved, he assumes that he must be at fault, since it is inconceivable to the mind of a young child that his mother or father, who gave him life, should not love what they gave him. Once a child doubts himself, it is not difficult for his parents to convince him that he is bad if he harbors angry or negative feelings toward them. If being good earns him love, the child will do everything in his power to be good, including suppressing "bad" feelings. Thus, guilt will lock him into a lifelong pattern in which he denies negative or hostile feelings toward those he is supposed to love. The unconscious holding back of such feelings produces a state of chronic tension in the muscles, especially of the upper back.

One other dimension in the feeling of guilt that John's case illustrates is its relation to sexuality. John felt guilty about his sexual involvement with a younger woman. Raised to believe that adultery was a sin, he could not fully accept that sexuality is an expression of love. Yet sexual excitement can pervade the whole body to the point where it even touches the heart. When this happens, contact anywhere between the two bodies has an erotic quality, although the charge is strongest at the erotic zones. As more of the body participates in the discharge of the excitation, the pleasure and satisfaction of orgasm are increased. With total body participation, one has a full orgasm that embraces the heart. Such an orgasm approaches the ecstatic.

Unfortunately, such a response is rare. For most men, the sexual climax is limited to ejaculation. For many women, climax does not occur. When it does, it is similarly limited to the clitoris. Climaxes vary, and it is fair to characterize them as full-hearted, halfhearted, or with very little heart. But this description of how individuals respond in sex applies to other activities, as well. In today's business world the head is more important than the heart. We are not wholeheartedly involved in our work, which in most cases is not a labor of love. What has the heart to do with making money? When work was an intense physical activity, more of our being was committed to it. To become emotionally involved in a business deal is a sure way to lose. In effect, what we have done is to isolate the three major segments of our bodies and our personalities. The head and the genitals have nothing to do with the heart or with each other. The head is for making money, the genitals for making whoopee, and the heart—the poor heart—has lost its connection to the world because it has been isolated from the head and the genitals.

Tensions in the voluntary muscular systems are under the control of the ego, which often countermands the heart's desire and creates an opposition between the head and the heart. Fearful of rejection, one stops reaching out with the hands to touch, the arms to hold, the lips to kiss, the mouth to suck (as a baby does), and the eyes to see. Those movements are restricted or inhibited by tensions in the shoulder girdle, the neck, and the jaw. Tension in the shoulders, as we have seen, stems from the need to suppress the impulse to strike out in anger or rage. A tight-mouthed, thin-lipped expression signifies distrust and disapproval of affection, the tight jaw denoting a determination not to give in to the longing for love, for closeness and contact, out of fear of disappointment or rejection.

A similar phenomenon occurs in the lower half of the body, caused by a ring of tension around the pelvis. This tension develops early in life from the experiences of shame, fear, and guilt about sexual feelings and their expression. We shall discuss this problem more fully in the next chapter. Suffice it to say at this point that the child learns he can be deeply hurt if he surrenders to his sexual desires and impulses. He cannot stop sexual excitation from occurring because it takes place on a level below conscious control. He can, however, block the melting of the self by the heat of passion, which constitutes the true surrender to love. This is accomplished by muscular spasticities in the lower back and pelvis that prevent the downward flow of excitation into the belly and genitals. Once that happens, sex has no connection to the heart, just as the heart has no connection to the mind.

The unity of the body is maintained on the deep, biological level; the split described above affects our conscious self, destroying the sense of being all of a piece, of integration, of wholeness. In such a situation, consciousness of the self is confined to the head, the seat of the ego. The "I" residing in the brain still possesses a heart and genitals but does not identify with them, because when one lives in the head, the body is regarded as an instrument of the I, or the ego. In this state of affairs, sexual activity becomes a performance designed

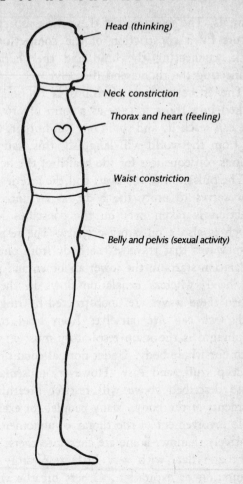

Head (thinking)

Neck constriction

Thorax and heart (feeling)

Waist constriction

Belly and pelvis (sexual activity)

Figure 6. The functional splitting of the body, isolating the heart

to demonstrate masculine or feminine prowess. It is not experienced as an expression of love.

This functional splitting of the unity of the body, shown in figure 6, separates the awareness of the head and its functions from the feelings in the heart and from the sexual activity in the genitals. The separation of these three aspects of the personality occurs by a constriction of the connecting passageways: the neck, connecting the head and the thorax; and the waist, connecting the thorax and the pelvis.

The effect of these divisions is to isolate the heart. It is locked in a thoracic cage as a form of protective custody. No one can reach it, and so no one can hurt it. Since a heart so cut off from the world will languish, this state of affairs can have serious consequences for the health of the heart.

The pulsation of the heart and the arteries is one of the forces that serves to unify the body on an unconscious level. That function is taken over on the conscious level by breathing, which is also a pulsatory activity. The respiratory movements form waves that traverse the body from one end to the other. Inhalation starts in the lower abdomen and proceeds upward to the head, whereas exhalation flows in the reverse direction. When these waves are unobstructed by rings of tension in the body, we can *feel* ourselves from head to toes. While the diaphragm is the main respiratory muscle, we actually breathe with our whole body. Under normal conditions, such breathing is deep, full, and easy. However, muscular tensions such as those described above will restrict breathing to one or two segments of the body. Many people, for example, breathe with little involvement of the thorax or abdomen. Such breathing is relatively shallow. Some are chest breathers; their abdomens are tight and flat, with very little respiratory movement during inspiration or expiration. Others breathe with the diaphragm and belly while the chest is rigid and immobile. These patterns become accentuated under stress, often resulting in sensations of distress. As we shall see later, such breathing can adversely affect the heart.

CHAPTER 2

Sex and the Heart

That sexual activity can have a powerful effect on the heart cannot be denied. Most adults have experienced a rapid increase in heartbeat at the moment of climax. Masters and Johnson[1] have reported rates as high as 130 beats per minute. One might think that this rapid heart rate is due to the strenuous physical activity of coitus, but there is nothing strenuous about making love. Since it is not normally a situation of conflict, it should be free from stress. The increased heart rate must be due, therefore, to the high level of excitement that develops just prior to and at the moment of orgasm. Because any high degree of emotional excitement increases the heart rate, this reaction is perfectly normal. If the heart rate does not increase at climax, it indicates that the level of excitement at discharge was low and limited to the genitals. Of course, if one doesn't reach a climax in intercourse, the heart would not react in the above fashion.

Studies suggest that the failure to reach a climax or to

experience emotional satisfaction in sex can have a deleterious effect on the heart. One study compared the sexual lives of 100 women, aged forty to sixty, who were hospitalized for an acute myocardial infarction with a control group of 100 women of the same ages who were hospitalized for other illnesses. Sexual frigidity and dissatisfaction were found among 65 percent of the coronary patients compared to 24 percent of the controls. These figures are statistically significant and indicate that a lack of sexual satisfaction should be considered a risk factor for heart disease in women.

Abramov[2] accepted a definition of frigidity as "a partial or complete inability to achieve orgasm." He classified women as frigid when (1) they never enjoyed sexual intercourse; (2) they enjoyed coitus but failed to achieve orgasm, which left them disappointed and emotionally unsatisfied; or (3) they had achieved orgasms in the past but lately had neither enjoyed coitus nor attained orgasm because of a husband's illness or impotence.

If there is a direct connection between sex and the heart in women, might not the same be true of men? Admittedly, the problem is different: The incidence of acute myocardial infarction is far greater among men, whereas the inability to reach a climax is relatively rare. Yet sexual dysfunction does exist among men. It often takes the form of impotence, which is the inability to become erect or to sustain an erection during intercourse. Just as frigidity undermines a woman's sexual pleasure, impotence limits the pleasure of sex for a man. It is thus fair to ask whether impotence bears any relation to heart disease.

In a study of male sexual dysfunction by Wahrer and Burchell, which examined 131 men, aged thirty-one to eighty-six, who had all been hospitalized for heart attacks, two-thirds were found to have experienced significant sexual problems in the weeks or months leading up to the attack. The authors of the study reported that 64 percent of the subjects were impotent, 28 percent had experienced a significant decrease (50 percent) in sexual frequency, and 8 percent suffered from premature ejaculation.[3] Impotence was not judged on the basis of one or two failures but only after weeks or months of unsuccessful attempts. Prematurity was determined by the patient's statement that he had reached a climax too quickly for his own satisfaction or for that of his partner. While there are no current figures on the incidence of male sexual dysfunction in the general population, the authors believe that these figures are higher than average.

If there is a relationship between sexual dysfunction and coronary heart disease, as this study suggests, is it a direct, causal relationship? There is no question that sexual dysfunction lowers a man's self-esteem and places him under stress. One woman said her husband "got very upset, swore, stamped around the room, got red in the face, beat his fist on the furniture and once or twice broke vases in response to his failure."[4] Such an outburst of rage could easily raise a person's blood pressure. Many men, though, would simply withdraw and blame themselves. Are these men subjecting their hearts to the same level of risk? The answer is yes, for as we shall see, it is the fullness of the discharge that ensures the health of the heart.

We might gain some clarity in this discussion if we use emotional satisfaction, not the ability to ejaculate, as the criterion for a healthy sexual response in men. Not all men who ejaculate or reach a climax are emotionally satisfied. Despite ejaculating, a man can feel sexually frustrated, just as a woman can. Men who ejaculate just prior to or immediately after penetration often feel dissatisfied. Other men, even if they are able to maintain an erection for some time, find that their ejaculation occurs without much feeling. It is unlikely that they feel emotionally satisfied with such a response.

But even emotional satisfaction is not ideal as a criterion for healthy sex. Many women report a feeling of warmth and satisfaction in just being held by a man. Sex is their avenue for contact and closeness, fulfilling a need left over from early childhood. For these women, the act of sex is less important than the sense of security that sexual intimacy provides. Men also use sex for purposes other than the expression of love. For many, it provides a narcissistic satisfaction by affirming their masculinity regardless of the quality of their sexual climax. These days, the same is true for many women, who see sexual contact as an affirmation of their sex appeal. However, when sex is used for ego purposes, it leaves the heart cold and uninvolved. Under these circumstances, coitus is not lovemaking but the acting out of various mixed feelings about the opposite sex, including some degree of sadism and contempt.

Yet there is some degree of love in nearly every act of sex. The genitals would not become charged and tumescent if blood did not flow from the heart—the organ of love—into the sexual organs. In most cases, however, the heart's participation is unconscious. It is functioning as a pump—mechanically. In such a state, the act of sex is rarely heartfelt. Sexual excitement is subdued, and the climax, if there is one, is lukewarm.

In the preceding chapter we saw that for many people the head, the heart, and the genitals do not operate together. Though this split affects every aspect of a person's behavior, it is nowhere more critical than in the act of sex. If a successful and competent businessman acts like a little boy at a party when he has had too much to drink, those around him might smile and explain it as a need to let go. However, when the same man is impotent with his wife, who dominates him as his mother did, and sexually excited by younger women, the situation is serious. The promise of love inherent in his marriage has given way to frustration and bitterness, which can end in major illness. Many women are in a similar position. Though they operate on the ego level as efficient professionals or business executives capable of commanding subordinates, in bed they need reassurance and are unable to reach a natural climax. Unfortunately, in such disturbed marital relationships, the children suffer even more than the adults, eventually undergoing the same splitting and dissociation of head, heart, and genitals from each other.

For an adult to be fulfilled, all of his being—his head, heart, and genitals—must enter into his important relationships. The fulfillment such wholeness brings is experienced most vividly in the kind of orgasms he enjoys. This concept of orgasmic fulfillment was propounded by Wilhelm Reich in 1924.[5] Reich observed that among his analytic patients, those who achieved such total orgasmic response were cured of their neurotic symptoms. Likewise, patients who did not achieve the capacity for full surrender in sex remained neurotic. Reich also found that this capacity distinguished healthy individuals in the general population. At the time he formulated this concept, Reich was an outstanding member of the analytic group around Freud in Vienna. However, his use of total orgasm as a criterion of emotional and mental health was rejected by his fellow analysts. How could such a criterion be useful, they asked, when they knew so many neurotic patients who had no complaints about their sexual life and regularly achieved orgasm? It became apparent to Reich that he and his colleagues defined the experience of orgasm in very different terms.

The analysts labeled every release by a woman, no matter how minuscule, and every ejaculation, no matter how little feeling was involved, an orgasm. Many people still speak of orgasm in the same way today, and many sexologists support their position, but to equate the experience of orgasm with the term *release* is to violate some deep, inner sense that an orgasm is something special. Reich had in mind the kind of response that involves the whole body in waves of pleasurable convulsions. At the peak of orgasm, the ego is overwhelmed and swept away by a flood of sensation. A deep sense of contentment, satisfaction, and well-being follows such a response. At night, a person falls asleep right after the climax; in the morning, he may feel rejuvenated and very much alive.

During a total orgasmic response, consciousness of the self

disappears in a fusion with the love object. Thus, love achieves its final goal, the union of the opposites. In many cases, there is also a feeling of unity with the pulsating universe. This latter feeling supports Reich's idea that in orgasm man feels his identification with cosmic processes. One woman said that she felt like a drop in the ocean. A man described his sensation as being among the stars.

One of my patients reported a similar experience, which happened the day his girlfriend announced that she wanted their relationship to end. At the news, my patient broke down in sobs and declared his love for her. She responded affectionately, and they made love. At the climax, his breathing quickened and deepened, and his pelvis moved in harmony with his respiration and the surges of his ejaculation. Waves of pleasurable discharge flowed through his body. He felt one with his lover and with the world. When it was over, he experienced a deep peacefulness and contentment. The next day, he was aware of an unusual sensation. His heart felt so open that he believed he could feel the beating of other hearts. The experience was so fulfilling that he longed to repeat it. At the time of this report, he had been unable to do so, although he and his girlfriend remained together.

This report is unusual in its recital of the effect on the heart of full orgasm. This patient said he was in love with his girlfriend before this event, but his love was guarded out of a fear of loss. His defense against being hurt was not to surrender body and soul. Strangely, it was the threat of loss that broke down his defenses, releasing a flood of longing and hurt. Once the worst had happened, he had nothing more to lose and could yield fully to his love. This is not unusual. How often people feel the depth of their love after they have lost the loved person! When the neurotic structure breaks down, the heart opens to love. In the sexual surrender the heart is fulfilled in love and opens to all of life.

For this patient, as for so many other people who have had

similar experiences, sexual fulfillment of this order transcends orgasm. It is what we dream of when we are young—the ecstasy and fulfillment of love. It is a tragic fact of life that those who experience it do so rarely. Even more tragic is that many people never experience it at all. Our hearts yearn for love, but the physical surrender to it is too frightening. We dare not surrender to the divine madness of love because our egos are too insecure to relinquish control. This control, our defense against being hurt, is accomplished by tensing our muscles, especially the chest muscles close to the heart. Such "armoring," as Reich called it, closes us off from the world and reduces the intensity of our interactions.

We have equated the heart with love and said that it is the seat of Eros. The desire for erotic contact flows with the blood, the carrier of Eros. As we've noted, the erotic areas of the body are characterized by the richness of their blood supply. When two such areas come in contact in a kiss or a sexual embrace, the erotic excitement is strong. However, kissing alone doesn't lead to orgasm. Its function is to increase the excitement, not to discharge it. Discharge is a function of movement. In the act of sex that movement has two phases.

The first phase covers the period from penetration to the beginning of climax. During the first phase the genitals are excited, that is, tumescent with blood, but they are not overexcited or ready for discharge. The partners build their excitement through the friction of the penis with the labia minora as the man's pelvis thrusts forward and the woman's reaches forward to receive him. As they pull away but not apart, the labia minora, like the lips they are, suck the penis. In this phase, the movements are voluntary and controlled. The breathing is deep and regular. Excitation builds in the pelvis and genitals until it can no longer be held. At this point, the second phase begins, leading to orgasm: There is a deep letting go as the discharge occurs, which is often accompanied by a sigh or cry as a powerful wave of expiration moves through the body.

With this wave the pelvis moves forward spontaneously, and orgasm is underway. The pelvis may make a number of involuntary moves sometimes very rapidly, sometimes more slowly, in rhythm with the breathing. In the male, the ejaculation takes place during this time and is part of the discharge. In older men in whom the emission of sperm has stopped, the ejaculation is greatly reduced to some seminal fluid, but the convulsive orgasmic response in the body remains the same.

The satisfaction of sex stems not from the voluntary movements but from the involuntary ones. Allowing these movements to occur requires a surrender of control. Since it is involuntary, the ejaculation provides some release for the man. The woman can have a similar climax through the involuntary contractions of the labia minora. However, as important as these movement are, they constitute a limited response, since they are confined to the genitals. When the involuntary movements embrace the pelvis, they provide a deeper feeling of pleasure and satisfaction; when the entire body participates, the orgasm is total. However, if these involuntary movements are inhibited, the fullness of the discharge is limited. Such inhibition occurs on an unconscious level.

An analysis of the body's structure shows that the major muscles of the body, those that effectuate movement and maintain the posture erect, are along the back of the body, extending into the extremities. Movement occurs when a charge travels along the back of the body, either up toward the head and arms or down toward the pelvis and legs. Reaching out with the arms for food or for an embrace occurs when this muscular charge flows up the back of the body. Reaching out with the pelvis in the sexual act occurs when the charge flows down the back. I have labeled this charge, or flow of excitation, *aggression*. In contrast, the flow of excitation from the heart, which I have labeled *longing,* is experienced as a wave along the front of the body. (Figure 7.)

Figure 7. The flow of excitation and feeling in the body

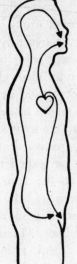

Flow of feeling along the back of the body = aggression (motor drive to reach out, strike out, move toward or away from)

Flow or feeling along front of the body = longing (desire for contact)

The flow of excitation up the front of the body can be experienced as longing by reaching out with the lips like a baby reaching for the breast of his mother. The feeling is intensified by reaching out with the arms at the same time. The downward flow resembles the sinking sensation in the belly that occurs when an elevator starts its descent too suddenly or what children experience in swings. It is experienced during sex, as the excitation moves down into the genitals, as a warm and melting feeling in the pit of the belly.

It is not uncommon for the upward flow along the back to be experienced as a surge of anger. If strong enough, it will move over the top of the head and into the eyes and teeth. At this point the teeth will be bared and the eyes ablaze with anger. The downward flow, meanwhile, is the force that drives the pelvis forward. The flow of excitation travels around the buttocks, along the pelvic floor, and into the genitals.[6]

In sexual activity, both of these components play a part. We feel a desire for closeness and erotic contact and a drive to possess, to merge with the partner. The desire for erotic contact is tender. The drive to merge is strong. The tenderness increases the excitation, and the aggressive drive seeks to discharge it. There is nothing sadistic about this drive for discharge. Without it there would be no fulfillment. However, without Eros, the tender component, there would be little excitation to discharge, and sexual activity would be devoid of real pleasure.

In the split personality, tenderness is associated with the child within, while the aggressive drive is associated with the adult ego. Such a person can experience either tenderness or aggression but not both at the same time. When childlike aspects dominate the personality, the person may be tender, sensitive, and even sensual but show little or no drive to achieve discharge and fulfillment. In sex the climax, should it occur, is pleasant but not urgent. It may even be accompanied by sadness, since it terminates the desired closeness and contact. For such people, contact is more important than release. In some cases, sex is carried on for long periods of time simply to maintain the contact, and the climax, which cannot be considered a true orgasm, is relatively low-keyed. A relationship between two such partners may be loving, but it is childish, not adult. On the other hand, when the adult aspect dominates the personality and behavior, the drive to possess the partner and to discharge is so strong that it leaves little time for tenderness. Sex becomes a performance with little feeling and no real satisfaction.

Tenderness is a function of softness. The rigid, narcissistic personality who operates by exercising his will is physically unable to feel any real tenderness. Because he is so rigid, any sexual excitement he feels travels through his body to his genitals, setting up a powerful tension that he seeks to relieve as soon as possible. For men, the ejaculation serves this purpose and thus feels good in the same way as any release from a tense or painful state. Since it doesn't provide the real pleasure and satisfaction that sex can offer, it leaves a man cold in his feelings toward his partner. The basic problem is the man's fear of full surrender to a woman. This fear is unconscious, but it is readily perceived in the bodily rigidity that blocks the natural convulsive movements of orgasm.

The fear of surrender to a woman is most characteristic of the "macho" man who identifies his manhood with erective potency. Reich noted that a

> severe disturbance of genitality . . . was especially true of those men who bragged the loudest about their sexual conquests and about how many times a night they "could do it." There was no doubt they were erectively very potent, but ejaculation was accompanied by little or no pleasure; or even the opposite, by disgust and unpleasant sensations.[7]

Other men have a masochistic attitude, which also affects their sexual or orgasmic response. These men view their sexual role as helping their partners achieve climax. As one man said, "I get my kicks when a woman comes." His own climax was relatively flat and weak. Whatever excitement he felt initially was drained out by the need to inhibit his discharge so that he could "be there" for the woman.

A man's fear of surrender to a woman has its roots in his early relationship with his mother. Giving in to his desire for a woman makes him as vulnerable to rejection and abandonment as he was when a little child. His defense is to hold in those feelings and to maintain some sense of security by denial and rigidity. He can only allow strong genital sensations to arise if they are dissociated from his heart. Sex without love gives him a sense of power that enables him to deny his fear of women, but sex without love is neither deeply pleasurable nor fulfilling.

In many ways, a woman's sexual problems are the opposite of a man's, but they have the same effect on her orgasmic potency. Her orgasmic response, when full and complete, is exactly the same as a man's in its convulsive movements, its total discharge of excitement, and its feelings of pleasure, satisfaction, and fulfillment. That kind of response depends on her ability to surrender fully to her love for a man, but it becomes difficult, if not impossible, when she harbors suppressed feelings of anger toward men, most of which stem from her relationship with her father. Marie Robinson[8] has shown that accepting and expressing these suppressed feelings of anger have enabled many "frigid" women to achieve a climax in the sexual act.

One of my own patients had always yielded to her husband's wishes in their sexual life, regardless of her feelings. When this matter came up in her therapy, I encouraged her to express her own feelings. She came back to me and said, "I said no to my husband for the first time. The next day I was surprised to find that I had a strong desire for sexual union, and when we made love, I had an orgasm."

For men, the act of love is rarely experienced as submission. Instead, men resist surrender by having power or being in control, both of which act as a defense against vulnerability and helplessness. By denying these feelings, they deny their fear of abandonment. Of course, they cannot protect themselves for long by playing power games, since such games undermine their relationships and end in the very loss of love they feared. When that happens, their helplessness, vulnerability, and hurt surface, and the power they thought they had reveals itself as an illusion.

In the final analysis, to surrender in love is not to surrender to another person but to one's self, one's heart and one's desire for love. Doing so, however, includes all one's feelings. When the ego relinquishes its hegemony, it gives up control over the body and its feelings. It must accept the fear of abandonment, the pain of loss, the anger of betrayal. It must also accept the self as helpless in all the major events of life: birth, love, sickness, death. But our helplessness in these areas does not leave us devoid of resources. Nature has provided human beings with the means to react and respond to insults and traumas. Our bodies have the capacity to heal themselves, as do our spirits. We can cry when we are hurt, become angry when we are betrayed, and fight or flee when we are threatened. These responses maintain our integrity so that we can cope effectively with the vicissitudes of life. Only when they are blocked do we become handicapped. Such blocking occurs in childhood and is caused by the very people to whom we look for protection and support in the critical years of our dependency. In the end we must submit to that crippling in the interest of survival. As we have seen in chapter 1, it takes the form of chronic muscular tensions in the chest and pelvis that reduce the body's mobility and responsiveness.

Such tensions, when locked in the pelvis, cause the man to "come" too quickly and the woman to "come" too slowly, blocking that lovely fusion that occurs when orgasm is simultaneous in both partners. It is mainly tensions and spasticities in the muscles of the lower back that immobilize the pelvis against the spontaneous movements of orgasm. We are familiar with these tensions from common complaints of lower back pain and discomfort. Since the pelvis rotates on the two hip joints, tensions in the muscles of the thigh, especially the quadriceps femoris, also act to restrict its mobility. All of these tensions are designed specifically to reduce sexual feeling, but they do not necessarily reduce excitement in the genitals, which is only a small part of one's sexual response. As a result, the sexual act becomes an act to relieve tension and not an expression of love.

Unlike tension in the chest, pelvic tension is not directly related to the fear of abandonment but to the trauma connected with the child's early sexual feelings. These develop between the ages of three and six years. The child experiences a strong sexual excitement in relation to the parent of the opposite sex. This excitement is a total body response (in other words, a true sexual feeling) with very little genital excitation and no focus on genital activity. Typically, the years from three to six, known as the Oedipal period, are a time of conflict with the parent of the same sex, who is often jealous if the other parent pays special attention to the child. That occurs quite often as parents use their children in their power struggles with each other and for the satisfaction of their own narcissistic needs. Thus, many a father is quite excited by his little daughter's admiration and sexual interest. It makes him feel manly and compensates for his wife's denigration of him. Frequently, the father's excitement has sexual undertones, which the little girl senses and which serve to heighten the charge between them. Mothers often behave similarly with their young sons. Although the phrase "A boy for you, a girl for me" may sound cute, in practice it proves to be less innocent. In fact, as many patients of mine have realized, parents are often unwittingly seductive with their children, inviting them into emotional and physical intimacies in which sexual feelings are only thinly disguised. We must also recognize that overt sexual activity of one kind or another between parents and children is not rare.

Let us examine in some detail what happens when a mother places her son in the difficult position of being her favorite or her intimate. Not surprisingly, the boy responds to his mother's attentions with increased desire and feeling, which alienates him from his father, whose affection and support he needs. His immature ego believes that he is superior to his father: Why else would his mother prefer him? This boy's attitude angers his father, who turns against him and holds him responsible for the situation. The mother cannot protect the child from the father's hostility, since to do so would further intensify the conflict. Besides, she has her own guilt feelings (generally unconscious) about her behavior with the boy. Faced with this situation, the boy wishes his father would die but at the same time is terrified that his father might kill him. Freud described this situation as Oedipal because it parallels the legend of Oedipus, who unknowingly killed his father and married his mother.[9] For the child, the situation is simply too frightening to face. In self-defense, he must cut off his sexual feelings for his mother to avoid any confrontation with his father.

Since such a move reduces the boy's orgasmic potency, it amounts to psychological castration. To cut off one's feelings is not the same as dismissing a thought from one's mind, since feelings are perceptors of bodily events. To cut off feeling, the body must be partially immobilized. Total immobilization is death. As noted above, tensions in the lower back, the thighs, and the pelvis serve to reduce sexual feeling.

The situation is identical for little girls who become sexually involved with their fathers, whether the involvement is acted out or not. The triangle that develops between the daughter, her father, and her mother is every bit as intense. Mother and daughter are rivals, and unconsciously each wishes the other were out of the way. But the girl, despite her favored position, cannot count on the support of her father, since it would increase her mother's jealousy. Her father, meanwhile, is immobilized by feelings of guilt stemming from his sexual involvement with his daughter. To protect herself, the young girl must cut off her sexual feelings for her father, which is accomplished by some degree of immobilization but even more by a ring of tension around the waist. Such a ring, which breaks the connection between the two halves of the body, is the typical feminine response to the problem rather than the rigidification that characterizes the masculine response.

For the child to resolve his Oedipal conflict by cutting off his sexual feelings for the parent of the opposite sex leads inevitably to a split in the personality by erecting a taboo in the mind of the child against giving in sexually to the person he—or she— loves best. As an adult, it becomes difficult to love one's sexual partner with all one's heart because such love is identified with the taboo parent. Many Victorian marriages suffered a crisis when men found themselves impotent with their wives but fully capable of having intercourse with a mistress or prostitute. Some Victorians solved this problem by accepting the practice of having lovers and mistresses as long as it was not made public. We see less of this problem now that the double standard has been discredited, but the taboo still operates on a deeper level. Men may have sex with their wives, but the act is often without passion and so without much love. The love one feels for one's wife takes on the quality of a duty. In time, even this routine sexual coupling loses all excitement, and we find men who are impotent with their wives.

In chapter 1 we discussed the case of John, a married man with grown children who fell in love with a younger woman and discovered that what he believed was impotence due to age vanished overnight when it was replaced by passion for his new partner. We noted, too, that John still professed to love his wife but that she had become like his mother in his eyes. Needless to say, one doesn't have sex with one's mother. It was a painful and tragic situation for John, who wished he could feel the same excitement with his wife. He was a victim of the incest taboo, having resolved his Oedipal conflict by cutting off all sexual feelings for his mother.

For a woman, the problem takes on a different form though the outcome is the same. She remains tied to her father as "Daddy's little girl" and cannot give herself fully to another man. Though she accepts her husband sexually, she feels no passion for him. Her response is limited to two roles in relation to her husband: Either she is the charming, seductive little girl, or she is the mother. These are roles she played with her father, as well, probably with some success. What she doesn't realize is that by acting like her husband's child or mother, she makes it impossible for him to see her as a sexual woman. Is it any wonder that there is so little fulfillment in marriage and that so many marriages fall apart?

In a general sense, it is fair to say that women are more identified with love feelings, whereas men are more identified with sexual feelings. By the same token, for a woman, love doesn't invariably mean sex, while for a man sex doesn't invariably mean love. When a woman gives herself sexually to a man, she generally regards it as an act of love, but her partner may refuse to see it that way to avoid the commitment that love implies. It is not commitment itself that he fears but the prospect of being trapped in a sexually unfulfilling relationship, as he was with his mother. To choose love would make him a mama's boy, whereas sex sets him free to pursue other women. The situation is the opposite for the woman. Long ago she became "Daddy's little girl," surrendering the independence that an identification with sexuality could provide.

To a degree, this difference in male/female responsiveness has lessened since the women's liberation movement. Yet it still exists. Since Eve, woman has been seen as the temptress and blamed for the fall of man. If she is seduced, it is her fault. Many young girls have been called sluts, whores, or tramps by their mothers for responding to their father's interest. If a young girl of five sits on her father's lap and he gets an erection, she is the one to blame. She is pushed away as if she had done something terrible. As a result of childhood experiences like these, too many women still feel a deep sense of humiliation about their sexual feelings. In contrast, the young boy is rarely humiliated for his sexual interest in his mother. She may tell him that he is a bad or dirty boy to have such feelings, but she usually expresses some admiration of or pride in his potential virility. From his father he may sense an implied threat of castration, but even the fact that he is regarded as a rival enhances his interest in and identification with his genitality. Thus, his greatest fear, once he grows up, is the loss of erective potency, which evokes a sense of shame. Women never suffer from this anxiety, as they nearly always can carry out the sexual act. Their anxiety is that if they yield too easily or are too aggressive sexually, they will be regarded as loose. In the past, an illegitimate pregnancy was a mark of shame for a woman— and a sign of virility for a man.

Much of this has changed with the demise of the double

standard, the advent of the pill, the availability of abortion, and the acceptance of women into the masculine world. Yet in the process of gaining more independence, the split in the modern woman's personality has widened. Operating more from her ego than her heart, she has become more rigid, more driven to achieve, and more vulnerable to heart disease. If she now dissociates sex from love, it can only mean that the child within is more denied, that her heart is more isolated, and that sexual fulfillment is even more evasive.

The following case illustrates some of the problems of the modern woman.

A woman executive in her early sixties, whom we will call Irene, came to treatment for a depressive reaction following her demotion from a top position in a large corporation. She needed help and she knew it—not just because of her depression but also because of the presence of several risk factors for coronary disease. She was overweight, she smoked heavily, and her blood cholesterol level was dangerously high.

These problems were reflected in Irene's body. Since her chest was greatly inflated, her breathing was poor. She stood as if she were holding herself up by her raised shoulders, not by her legs. Her abdomen and pelvis were heavy and flabby. She tried to hold her belly in, but all she could do was to constrict her waist so that there was little connection between thorax and pelvis. Her legs were thin, and she had a problem with her feet that made standing and walking painful.

Irene was aware that she had self-destructive tendencies. She knew that smoking was harmful, and she had tried to stop through hypnosis, but it had worked for a very short time. Her personal physician urged her to lose weight, but she found dieting almost impossible. She admitted at one session, "Last night I went out and bought cookies and ice cream and ate it all, which I shouldn't have done." Poor Irene. She was really starved for pleasure. Both physically and emotionally, she was in bad shape.

The therapeutic approach to changing behavior is to help the patient understand the dynamics of the inner struggle and to express the feelings relating to that struggle. Irene was sad (she saw her life as a failure) and in pain. She had been divorced for a number of years and had raised a child alone. Her first need was to feel her sadness and to cry. In her effort to function in the modern business world on a par with men, she had suppressed most of her feelings. This was not too difficult to accomplish; I helped her breathe and then got her to kick the bed and say, "Why," which brought up some tears. She was surprised at how much better she felt after she cried. I also encouraged her to do some kicking at home on her bed and instructed her to lie prone on her back and to kick with extended legs. To kick is to protest, and Irene had much to protest about.[10]

Irene had been an only child and a very pretty one; naturally she was the apple of her father's eye, but he died when she was five years old. Her mother told her that she had to be a soldier like her father, which to the little girl meant to be brave and hold in her sadness. In a therapy session she remarked, "I've always known there was pain in me. There was a constriction in my throat, but I didn't connect it to my heart." At the time she said this, she was lying on the couch. I suggested she reach up with her hands and say, "Daddy, daddy." She did and burst into deep sobbing. "I've held in this pain all these years," she said afterward. "I didn't know where to put it."

Those early events had shaped the course of Irene's life and determined her fate. While the loss of her father during the Oedipal period was an important factor, other forces also played significant roles. Of these the most powerful was the sense of guilt she felt about her sexual feelings for her father. She regarded his death as a punishment for violating the incest taboo in her desire for him. She also feared her mother, the jealous rival, against whom she had no protection once her beloved father was gone. The effect of these early years were visible in her adult body and behavior. Not only was Irene still trying to be a brave soldier as her mother demanded, but she had also dissociated herself from her sexuality and was struggling to gain self-esteem through achievement and success. She felt obliged to hold herself up by the efforts of her will alone. To break down, to cry, was to face a depth of despair about the loss of her father that she could not tolerate.

Irene had been married twice and had been deeply in love two other times. Unfortunately, neither of her marriages was to men she loved, and neither of the men she loved offered to marry her. This script had been determined by the events of her childhood. In her unconscious mind, Irene equated the men she loved with her father, who had been taboo. Since the taboo continued to operate where deep love was concerned, she married men who did not evoke her strong passions. Her drive to be independent was an important part of her struggle, since it denied and countered a deeper wish to be taken care of. Her fear was that if she let herself be dependent and gave herself fully to a man, she would be abandoned, as she had been by her father. As a result, she married men on whom she could not depend and who required her care. Her first husband was unable to hold a steady job, and her second turned out to be a manic-depressive who required hospitalization. In marrying them, she managed to preserve her independence, or pseudoindependence. Yet by allowing them to use her, she felt trapped and depressed.

Holding herself up as she did, Irene could not let go to love or sex. Like many women, she gave herself sexually but in a fashion that was too submissive, too passive. Only rarely did she experience a climax during the sexual act. Without orgasm she had none of the release that sex can provide.

When Irene recognized in the course of therapy that she was being used by the man with whom she was then involved, her anger mounted. She hit the bed with a tennis racket to vent her anger at his betrayal. At the same time, she began to feel angry at all men, those who used her and those who left her. She even became angry at her father for having died at a time when she needed him.

The tension in Irene's back and around her shoulders was a clear indication of the amount of anger she held in. She literally had her back up. But her awareness of its existence and her willingness to express it helped Irene greatly. Ventilating her anger reduced her guilt and allowed her to give in to her sexuality more fully.

Irene was fortunate to be able to bring her anger to the surface before she fell seriously ill. Another patient of mine, whom we shall call Paul, was not so lucky. Paul first came to me for a consultation for his impotence seven years after he was divorced and nine years after he had suffered a heart attack. At the time of his attack, he was a typical Type A personality: competitive, driving, overworking, and overeating. He smoked, his cholesterol was up, and his blood pressure was climbing. Working all the time at two jobs, he had reached a state of absolute exhaustion. As fate would have it, the attack occurred just as he was ready to quit, convinced he had finally succeeded. However, the stress of his work was small compared with that of his home life.

Paul described his wife as a domineering woman who always got her own way. Over the years their love relationship deteriorated steadily, and sex between them became an occasional and relatively formal arrangement with no sparks. At the time of the attack, they rarely made love. Nevertheless, Paul remained faithful to his wife. More surprisingly, he never masturbated. He explained this by saying, "My father scared the hell out of me." Even when he did make love with his wife, Paul never ejaculated until after his wife had an orgasm. "I had to hold back a long time," he said. "I was masterful at holding back." It was during the latter part of his marriage that he became unable to maintain his erection.

Holding back was a necessity for Paul, for he knew he was short-tempered. He had learned this shortly after his marriage. One evening soon after he had returned from the war, Paul's mother-in-law, who was German, accused him of killing her relatives. Paul lost his head, went for his mother-in-law, and was strangling her when he realized what he was doing. After that incident he vowed never to lose control again—and he didn't. Despite many arguments with his wife, he never exploded.

Paul described his relations with his parents as follows: "I was close to my mother, and she spoiled me. My younger sister was my father's favorite. He and I were never friends and never discussed things. If I talked back to him, I got the back of his hand until, when I was sixteen, I beat him in a fistfight. After that he never touched me again. However, when I was a child, he used to punish me regularly by spanking and strapping. He said he was trying to make a man out of me." In some ways his father succeeded. Paul played all the competitive sports and went in for hunting and fishing. Throughout his life, he proved he could be tough. But he also had another side, which he had learned to suppress—a soft, tender side tied to a feeling of vulnerability.

When I asked him when he had last cried, Paul related an incident that had occurred about twenty years earlier. He had been an auxiliary policeman in the town where he lived. One day he was called to the scene of a car accident in which two small children were badly injured. The sight of their pain brought tears to his eyes. He also recalled sobbing at the news of his mother's death, and remembered, as a boy at camp, going off into the woods alone to cry. He was an unhappy child, and even as an adult, the unhappiness of little children could make him feel sad.

Paul's struggle was between the two sides of his personality: the tough, manly exterior and the soft, childlike, sad interior. To look at him, he seemed self-confident and relaxed. However, when he dropped his easy smile, his face took on a grim look of sadness, and in his eyes I saw a murderous rage. As far as his body went, he was well built and muscular, but he had a paunch that he wanted to lose. Pads of fat around his pelvis suggested a feminine aspect to his personality. His pelvis was tight and pulled back. The upper half of his body looked strong; the lower half, weak. This split between the upper and lower half of the body is commonly found in men who feel they have to be macho. But that very need to project a manly image stems from an inner feeling of inadequacy. True manliness lies in a person's identification with his sexual feelings, not in his sexual performance.

Paul's manliness had been undermined by his father, whose treatment of him as a boy amounted to psychological castration. That was the meaning of the tendency to a feminine configuration in his pelvis. The more serious trauma, however, was his mother's betrayal. One cannot know all the reasons why she failed to stand up for him and protect him from his father, but one of them had to be a sense of guilt about her seductive relationship with Paul. Paul himself was not aware that his closeness to his mother had provoked his father's jealousy and rage and that his mother had used him against his father. While Paul felt great anger at his father for the humiliating beatings he had suffered, he harbored an even greater rage against his mother. The murderous attack on his mother-in-law can only be understood as the projection of a long pent up anger at his mother for her seduction and betrayal. But Paul could never express his anger directly to his mother because he felt guilty about his sexual interest in her. Guilt also made him deny his hatred. Nevertheless, on some deep level, he continued to love his mother. Thus, like John, whose case we discussed in chapter 1, Paul became trapped in a love-hate ambivalence.

In time, he transferred all the ambivalent feelings he felt for his mother to his wife, who dominated him just as his mother had and to whom he was sexually submissive. How he must have hated his wife! But he held back and denied his hatred as well as the sadness and pain he felt at the loss of love. Eventually, guilt made him impotent. In the end, it was the heartbreak he felt and the anger he suppressed that were responsible for his heart attack.

In this chapter we have emphasized the importance of healthy sexuality in preventing a heart attack. It does so by keeping the chest soft and allowing the tension that builds up in the chest during the course of a competitive existence to be discharged naturally. Orgasm is like a rebirth, or, more literally, a rejuvenation. Not only are the muscles softened and relaxed, but this softening extends deep into the tissues of the body, including the arteries.

A full orgasm, one that leaves the body totally fulfilled, quiet, and contented, is a convulsive movement of the body in which the pelvis swings involuntarily with the breathing. The same convulsive movement occurs when a person sobs deeply. Each sob is a pulse or wave that flows through the body, bringing the pelvis forward as the wave reaches the pelvic floor. The sob is a vocal release superimposed on the expiratory wave. Between sobs there are short inspiratory gasps during which the pelvis moves backward. In deep crying the movement of the pelvis is involuntary, just as it is in orgasm. This similarity between the two reactions explains in part why many women burst into tears when they experience an orgasm. Their crying is an expression of paradise found and reflects the sadness of paradise lost. The orgasmic convulsion opens the path for such deep crying, which shares the same bodily movements. By the same token, when a person can give in to deep crying and allow the waves of sadness to flow through his body, he will also be able to give in to the convulsive movements of orgasm.

Unfortunately, for most people such a surrender is not easy. In the next chapter, we will examine the process of growing up in modern culture to find out why.

CHAPTER 3

At Heart We Are Still Children

Das kind ist alles herz.
German Proverb

Just as a woodsman can read the life history of a tree from a cross section of the trunk, so it is possible to read the life history of a person from his body. Growth in the human organism, though, proceeds in stages, not in years. Unlike the growth rings in a tree, these stages are not sharply demarcated, but we recognize them nevertheless because each has a special quality: the helplessness of babyhood, the inquisitiveness of childhood, and so forth. These stages are like layers, each of which remains alive and functioning in the adult person, adding their special quality to the whole.

The qualities that each stage or layer adds to life may be summarized as follows:

Baby	age 0–2	=	love and bliss
Child	age 3–6	=	playfulness and joy
Boy or girl	age 7–12	=	adventure, challenge
Youth	age 13–19	=	romance, ecstasy
Adult	age 20–	=	responsibility, fulfillment

The growth we are considering is the development and expansion of consciousness. Each layer represents different awareness of the self and the world. Consciousness, however, is not an isolated part of the personality. It is a function of the whole organism, an aspect of the living body. It develops in relation to the growth of the body physically, emotionally, and psychologically. It depends on experience, gains depth through the acquisition of skills, and becomes confirmed in activity.

Equating qualities of consciousness with stages of growth does not mean that each new dimension of the self arises fully formed within a certain age period. Playfulness actually begins in babyhood but does not become a conscious activity until childhood. Nor does it stop with childhood. To the degree that our growth is free and undisturbed, we retain an ability to play throughout life, though playfulness is not the dominant mode of our mature years, as it was in childhood. This is true of the other qualities listed as well. Adventure appeals to us throughout life, but if as adults we have accepted the responsibility of family, leadership, and a creative undertaking, our desire for adventure is subordinated to our more mature role.

But let us start at the beginning. The baby is characterized by a strong desire to be held and nourished by his mother. That desire is an expression of his love for her. Physical closeness between the two is more intimate in the act of nursing, which fulfills the basic biologic needs of both baby and mother. The fulfillment of the baby's need for contact and nurturance gives him a feeling of blissful contentment. Every feeling of love in an adult stems from this infantile layer in his personality. The desire for intimate contact (as found in nursing, kissing, genital embrace, etc.) determines every feeling of love. If a person is in touch with his heart, he is in touch with the baby within him. This may explain why babies so easily touch the heart of most individuals. To the degree that a person is cut off from the baby in his personality, he is blocked from experiencing the fullness of love. That can easily happen, as we shall see later, when a baby is deprived of needed closeness and warmth.

As an infant grows into a child, the need for continuous closeness gives way to a need to investigate the world now opening to him; to explore persons, things, space, and time so that he can construct a picture in his mind of reality. In this process, the child also explores his own being in relation to the world and develops a conscious sense of self. It is during childhood that the ego develops. It becomes a definitive structure at about the age of six to seven. Until that time reality is not perceived as fixed or final, and the child's imagination runs free. He can play at being a father, a mother, or even a baby. In his play and make-believe he learns the feel of life. Since the child is not aware of any serious consequences to his play, he can give himself wholeheartedly to it in all innocence. A child whose babyhood was fulfilled and who is now free to play undisturbed by adults feels a sense of joy. However, if the child's innocence is shattered by the intrusion of adult feelings and concerns, that joy turns quickly to sorrow.

A child reaches out with love to a broader world than that of a baby, whose world is limited to those immediately responsible for his well-being. In addition to the family, the child has friends whom he loves dearly. We know that children play house, doctor and patient, and other games in which they explore their bodies. Since sex is one of the realities of life, it, too, must be investigated in play if it is to be integrated into the child's understanding of the world. Children feel a great excitement in this sexual play, and although it is entirely innocent it is one type of play that adults often condemn. By projecting their own feelings onto children, adults introduce into their minds such concepts as shame and guilt and destroy the joy that these playful sexual activities offer. Once children become aware of sexuality, they inevitably become curious about the sexuality of the adults around them. Both the little girl with her father and the little boy with his mother experience the excitement of the sexual charge. But all this is still inno-cent, for it is primarily in the service of knowing the world. The wish of the little boy to marry his mother or of the little girl to marry her father is a make-believe activity. Parents who take it seriously either by responding or by disapproving do real harm to their children. To children, parents are always love objects, which does not preclude sexual feelings.

Childhood may be said to end when the child gains a coher-ent picture of his personal world and his own self. Having achieved this step, he begins to investigate the larger world outside the home and his circle of childhood playmates. School becomes a secondary center of activity, the place to learn about the real, objective world in contrast to the largely subjective world of the young child. The games young people play during these years are real, and the consequences are important; games allow them to test themselves against each other and at the same time teach them to cooperate in group activities. As skills are sharpened, hierarchies develop. One boy may be the best runner, another the best ball player, etc. Girls go through a similar process of rank formation. These young people are no longer innocent, but since they are unburdened by responsibili-ties, they are free to enjoy the challenges and excitement of preadolescence. Friendships are also deeper, and the love in-vested in them is more objective.

Adolescence begins with sexual maturity on a biologic level. The fire that has been smoldering so long bursts into a brilliant hot flame. It had flamed briefly during the Oedipal period, but those were fires made of kindling wood; now the logs are burning. The passion may be intense, but since emotional maturity lags behind, adolescents tend to idealize the love object. For them, the excitement of romantic love is over-whelming. The romanticism of youth combines the baby's de-sire for closeness, the child's playfulness, and the youngster's taste for adventure. What is lacking is a sense of responsibility for the serious consequences of love. When one is ready to assume those responsibilities, the stage of adulthood has been reached.

A healthy adult is the integrated total of the different stages: a baby at heart, a child in his imagination, a young boy in his spirit of adventure, and a young man in his romantic aspirations. As an adult, he is also aware of the consequences of his actions and is prepared to assume responsibility for them. However, if he has lost touch with the earlier layers of his personality, he will be a sterile, compulsive, and rigid person whose assumption of responsibility represents an imposed obligation rather than a natural desire.

Only those individuals fulfilled in each earlier stage reach adulthood with integrated personalities. If an earlier stage is not fulfilled, fixations result that bind part of the personality while the rest of the personality moves on, diminished, to the next stage. The personality becomes split: Though on one level a person may function like an adult, on another he behaves like a baby or a child. The most dramatic example of this split that I've encountered was a man in his forties who came for a consultation because he was still sucking his thumb. He held a responsible position and was the father of grown children, but in situations of stress he put his thumb in his mouth, hiding the action with his other hand. Another rather extreme example was a young woman in her late twenties who was having difficulties in her marriage. She dressed well and looked like a mature, intelligent person, but when she took off some of her clothes so that I could observe her body, she looked like an eleven-year-old girl. Her body was so markedly underdeveloped that it was not surprising that she would have problems in her marriage.

Personality has a dual aspect: one psychological and the other physical. In a healthy person the two are congruent. When they are not, it denotes some disturbance in the development of the personality. When a person is more intellectually advanced than he is emotionally mature, he will appear and act very sophisticated without the depth of feeling to support such an attitude. It is hard to find the reverse, where a person is emotionally mature but lacking understanding and common sense, because emotional maturity only develops when there is an understanding of life.

What happens when babies are deprived of the love, support, and nurturing they need? Here is a case report: Jim was a fifty-three-year-old man who came in for a consultation about some problems he was experiencing in a relationship with a younger woman. He said that he loved her very much and that she reciprocated his affection. However, she denied him the pleasure and satisfaction of sexual intimacy. They had been intimate when the relationship first began, but during the past two years there had been no sexual activity between them. Jim couldn't understand why, since she proclaimed her love for him and enjoyed being with him. He was also disturbed by a commitment he had made to support her as she developed her career, which proved to be an expensive commitment, although Jim could afford it.

One can easily guess at the reason for the lack of sexual responsiveness on the part of Jim's woman friend. She was being supported by a man considerably older than she. While there are many women who would not be disturbed by the implications of such a sexual relationship, this young woman could not deny its incestuous character. Jim was a father figure to her, but he couldn't see the problem in this light.

To counsel Jim, one had to understand him. There was no better way than to study his body. I began at his face, traditionally the most expressive part of the body. Jim's habitual facial expression was a cherubic smile. Far from a grimace of unfelt friendliness, it was the smile of a child. However, when Jim dropped the smile and let his face relax, he took on an expression of deep sadness, almost a look of despair. Jim didn't allow this expression to emerge often. In fact, he didn't even recognize it as his own. When he saw his face in a mirror with its sad look, he said, "I am a happy man. All my friends think of me as an upbeat person." It was true that he was someone who always saw the brighter side of things. That same quality was reflected in his voice, which had a higher pitch than the normal male voice.

Jim held up his spirits and also held up his body. His shoulders were raised, and his chest was elevated and held in an overinflated state. The appearance of his thorax suggested that he suffered from emphysema, a condition in which breathing is difficult and painful because the overinflation of the lungs has resulted in some destruction of lung tissue. Emphysema is generally associated with heavy smoking, but Jim wasn't a smoker and didn't have any symptoms of emphysema. When questioned about breathing problems, he said that he had suffered from asthma as a child but hadn't experienced any attacks during adulthood. However, his breathing was very shallow, with almost no movement in his chest.

The lower half of Jim's body looked weak and somewhat underdeveloped. His pelvis was narrow, and there was the same accumulation of fatty tissue around his genitals that one sees in fat little boys. His legs and feet looked too weak to support him well. All this pointed to a deep insecurity in his personality, which he compensated for by holding himself up by sheer force of will. It was no accident that his shoulders were raised and his voice high. For him to let down, to drop the pitch of his voice, lower his shoulders, and deflate his chest would have released an intolerable degree of sadness.

Jim's case is particularly relevant because he was overweight and suffered from a high level of cholesterol, which tended to stay in the range of 300 mg. despite medical treatment and changes in his diet. Given these risk factors as well as his inflated chest, Jim could have been considered a candidate for a heart attack. However, his was not the typical Type A personality despite the fact that he was successful in business and often worked very hard. His manner was easy going and laid back, at least on the surface, and he seemed neither to be subject to a sense of time urgency nor driven to achieve. He did say, however, that he wanted to be very rich because of what money could buy. He was to discover much later in analysis that it couldn't buy love from his girlfriend, although it did provide a false sense of security.

Where did Jim's insecurity come from? What was the basis of the sadness he struggled to deny? The answer to both questions lay in his body, especially in his overinflated chest, which was related to his asthma. Jim said that his first attack occurred at six months of age, although he had no recollection of it or any understanding of what might have caused it. I suggested to Jim that he might have suffered a trauma at that age and advised him to consult his father, who was still living, to see if he could shed some light upon the events of that time. My guess was that Jim had been nursed for six months and then weaned, which had constituted for him an overwhelming loss of his mother. I imagined further that after he had cried his heart out to no avail, he had sucked in air and held his breath to stop the crying in the interest of survival.

Jim was surprised and impressed when he asked his father about his infancy and the events surrounding the onset of his asthma and he learned that he had been breast-fed for six months and then weaned because his mother had become depressed. His father had no recollection of Jim's reaction to the weaning or any awareness of a connection between it and the onset of Jim's asthma. Not all babies react violently to being weaned. Some actually give up the breast voluntarily in favor of the bottle, generally because they don't find breast-feeding all that exciting or satisfying. Jim, however, reacted to the loss as if it were the end of the world. It is not uncommon for the breast to take on such significance for a baby. The loss of the breast, then, becomes a catastrophic event to which the baby responds by screaming and crying. The effort to restore that vital connection continues until the child is exhausted and has to stop for lack of energy. At this point the thoracic muscles are so contracted that the chest is locked in an inflated position.

As an asthmatic child, Jim did not participate in athletic activities, which may have accounted for the lack of development in his legs. In my opinion, however, emotional factors played a greater role. Jim described his mother as sickly and prone to depression and stated that as a child he felt that he had to take care of her. Her failure to provide the support and nurturing he needed forced him to hold himself up by his will, which he continued to do throughout adulthood. To let down would have brought up the feeling of abandonment that, it seemed, he had so valiantly overcome as a child. Could he survive reexperiencing the intolerable grief he had felt as an infant when he lost the breast? Jim never asked himself this question, but his body clearly indicated that he felt he could not afford to take the risk. But holding himself up and containing his grief posed another risk, namely, the possibility of a serious heart attack. Two years later Jim did suffer a heart attack following the death of a sister, to whom he was deeply attached.

Is there a connection between asthma and heart disease? Such a connection is worthy of research, especially since a disturbed respiratory function is common to all heart attack victims. Some time ago I was consulted by a man in his late forties who suffered from a severe asthmatic condition. He recognized the importance of emotional factors in his illness and was hopeful that therapy might ameliorate his condition. The breathing exercises he did during the consultation seemed to make him feel much better. However, because of a pending vacation, the beginning of his therapy had to be postponed for one month. He never kept his appointment. His wife called to say that he had suffered a fatal heart attack.

Fate took a hand in Jim's life, as it does in all our lives, for better or worse. Fifteen years before he came to see me, he suffered another great loss with the death of his beloved wife of twenty years. Jim was devastated by this event and experienced an agony that he thought he might not survive. He sat alone in his room for days, crying his heart out. The thought that he had to live for his two young children sustained him when he felt that he could no longer endure the pain. Then, slowly, his pain diminished, and he resumed a normal life. He married again a few years later, but his second wife suffered from severe depression, and the marriage ended in divorce two years later. When I met him, he was involved in another unsatisfying relationship, as we have seen.

Another patient of mine, a forty-year-old woman named Marta, suffered from depression.[1] Her body, like Jim's, revealed some of the reasons for her depression. The upper half of her body was held up as if by conscious effort; her shoulders were raised, and her chest was high and inflated. Her abdomen and pelvis, meanwhile, were tight and drawn in. Her legs were rigid and thin, the leg muscles so contracted that her legs looked like sticks. It appeared that she had little feeling in her legs and that they functioned merely as mechanical supports. This lack of support, which pointed to a deep feeling of insecurity, could be accounted for by the fact that she, like Jim, had suffered a trauma in early life. That trauma was a break in the loving connection to her mother, which, as we shall see, first occurred when Marta was two months old. The effect of that break was to undermine Marta's sense that her mother would be there for her. This insecurity became transferred to mother earth, giving rise to the feeling that even the ground would not be there for her. No wonder her legs were undeveloped. Marta had to hold herself up by her shoulders because she couldn't feel the ground with her feet.

Marta reported the following:

> Until I was two months old, my mother and grandmother would rock me and nurse me until I went to sleep. Then one day my mother decided that I was now grown up and this indulgence should stop. When I cried, she left me alone to let me cry myself out. I cried for hours. My grandmother went crazy, but

my mother refused to let her go into my room to pick me up. Finally, I stopped crying, and my mother said, "See." They opened the door and saw I was blue. I had vomited and was choking on the vomitus.

Marta related similar horrors from her childhood—stories her mother told with pride.

When crying is serious enough to pose the threat of asthma or choking, it is no wonder that the child suppresses it, along with the longing to reach out for love. Tightening the throat blocks the impulse to cry; holding back the shoulders blocks the impulse to reach out. By tightening the chest wall as well, one effectively blocks any feeling of pain and sadness from reaching consciousness. Both Marta and Jim showed unmistakable signs of having done just that, but while Marta was seriously depressed, Jim was not. His support of himself was more effective than hers, for despite her raised shoulders, Marta could not keep up her spirits, perhaps because her mother was cruel, while Jim's was simply unavailable.

The rigidity of the chest wall described above constitutes what Reich called "armoring." Like the breastplate worn by knights of old to protect the heart against a spear or arrow, its purpose is to protect the individual against the danger of having his heart pierced by the arrow of love. To pierce that defense would free long-suppressed feelings of anguish. The well-armored person unconsciously feras that he will find himself in the same situation he was in as an infant or child—unable to breathe because of the pain and anguish. The child—and later the adult—feels panic at his inability to get enough air. Underneath the panic is the fear of death by suffocation.

Such is the crisis that the baby suffers at the loss of his mother. Generally the baby survives the loss, but nothing is resolved. Although the crisis may pass, the fear of abandonment, the associated feeling of panic, and the pain of unfulfilled longing persist in the unconscious—in many cases, not far below the surface. Suppressing these feelings may inspire a sense of security, but if the longing for love is awakened, the underlying feelings of abandonment and panic will be activated. No wonder such a person is afraid to open his heart fully and to reach out for love.

If crying is the primary release mechanism for feelings of heartbreak, not crying is the primary defense. The unconscious inhibition of crying is accomplished mainly by holding the breath. When a person comes to therapy for some emotional disturbance such as depression or anxiety, it is important to get him to breathe more deeply. As long as he or she breathes shallowly, any discussion of the person's problems remains an intellectual exercise and doesn't touch on deeper feelings. One of the ways to help a person breathe more deeply is to have him lie over what I call the bioenergetic stool (fig. 8). The backward stretch that the stool provides opens the chest and stimulates the respiratory process.

The following case illustrates the use of the stool in deepening breathing and thereby calling forth the feelings associated with the loss of love. A young woman named Ruth whose complaint of depression and anxiety brought her to therapy was

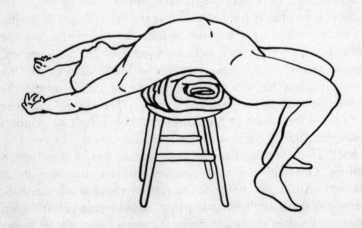

Figure 8. The bioenergetic stool

lying over the stool with the instruction to breathe easily and freely. She did so for a minute or two, then suddenly cried out in a gasping voice, "I can't breathe. I can't breathe." With these words, she rose from the stool, collapsed onto the floor, and broke into the deepest crying. What had happened was this: The deeper breathing had awakened her longing, touched her sadness, and opened the floodgate of her tears. However, when she attempted to block this flood of feeling by choking off her sobs, she also choked off her air, which caused her to panic. Fortunately, the flood of tears was too strong to resist, and she broke down and cried deeply, which released the pain and allowed her to breathe more fully.

The story Ruth told afterward was most revealing. She was the firstborn of fraternal twins and was the stronger of the two. The mother nursed both, which was a difficult undertaking, since both babies wanted to nurse at the same time. Ruth was more aggressive, which provoked an angry response from her mother, who considered her a monster. Furthermore, the two girls were locked in an intense sibling rivalry not only for their mother's affection but later for their father's. Ruth was rejected in both of these relationships, which hurt her deeply.

We have seen that the first stage of life, babyhood, is for many people not a period of fulfillment but one of deprivation. Some experience a loss of love that has devastating effects on the personality. In most cases, however, the experiences of babyhood will not prevent a child from reaching out in all innocence for the love he so desperately needs. During the Oedipal period, he will reach out to the parent of the opposite sex.

It is during the second stage of growth, childhood, that the child becomes keenly aware of his sexuality, thanks in part to a temporary increase in the production of sexual hormones during this period. But the young child who reaches out with sexual feelings to the parent of the opposite sex is seeking a loving connection, not a genital one. In this activity, as in so many others, the child is playing at being genital.

An understanding of the subtle dynamics in the relationship between parents and children during the Oedipal period is essential to a comprehension of the problems that emerge in adult life. I have emphasized the child's need for love, but of only slightly lesser importance is his need for recognition. Between the ages of three and six, the child gains a conscious sense of self. By the age of six he acquires an identity that tends to endure with small changes throughout life. This process is related to the growth and development of the ego, which is largely completed in its essential aspects during this period. A person's identity is intimately connected to his sexual nature. A child is very conscious that he (or she) is either a boy or girl and is keenly aware that his role and position in life will be determined by his sex. This is the pattern of normal development, but it depends on whether the child is seen, recognized, and accepted as a sexual person by both parents. If he is, the child's identity becomes solidly rooted in his sexuality. As an adult, the person's identity is grounded in who he is and not based on what he does.

Unfortunately, in too many families that respectful recognition of the child as a sexual person is lacking. Too often, boys and girls are humiliated for any overt manifestation or expression of sexual feeling. At the same time, they are covertly seduced into some expression of sexual feeling for which they will be humiliated. Oedipal problems would not exist if parents did not use children for their personal needs and games. Some seek sexual excitement from their children to make up for their own lack of feeling; others seek closeness and intimacy because of their inner loneliness. Many parents want their children to fulfill their own dreams, to be successful where they failed, or simply to support their image of themselves as good and proper parents. In all these maneuvers the child's independence and individuality are subverted.

To use a child in this fashion, a parent has to make him feel guilty. Parents have many ways of instilling guilt in a child, but they all filter down to guilt about sexuality. The reason for this is that sexuality is associated with freedom and independence. Undermine independence and you undermine sexuality, and vice versa. Few individuals in our culture are free from some guilt about their sexuality, although this guilt is unconscious in most cases and is manifested only in an inability to surrender fully to sexual feeling.

Parents as well feel guilty about sexuality, a feeling they deny and rationalize as morality and respectability. But a morality based upon guilt is not a true morality. Not all "respectable" people have kept to the straight and narrow path of virtue, and they assuage their feelings of guilt by projecting them onto their children. Other feelings can also influence a parent's attitude toward a child's sexuality. Envy and jealousy can turn a parent against a child's innocent pleasure in his sexuality. Some parents' attitude can be expressed as "I wasn't allowed to enjoy my sexuality, and you cannot have what I didn't have." We would be blind if, as students of human nature, we didn't see the covert and often overt hostility that exists between some parents and their children. More often than not, this hostility can be traced back to the parent's feelings about their own sexuality—feelings that were instilled in them long ago by their own parents.

How do these childhood experiences affect the individual as he grows up and moves out of his home and into the world? The answer to this question can be found in analytic work with patients. Analyzing the origin of a patient's fear of love and closeness, of openness and directness, always brings one back to the events of childhood. Analysis is necessary because very few patients remember these early events. In fact, most people have few memories of the early years of their life, even though those early events, since they were most vividly experienced, should provide the most vivid memories. This amnesia about early life experiences was well known to Freud and the other analysts of his time. If such memory loss were due to a physiological disturbance, no recall would be possible. But through analysis and through working with the body, many significant events of childhood can be brought back to consciousness.

In psychogenic amnesia, as Arthur P. Noyes calls this phenomenon, "the absence of memory is an active, defensive process; the patient refuses to remember . . . Consciousness is protected from unpleasant or inconvenient memories."[2] Such memory loss denotes an unconscious denial of reality. This conclusion is supported by the observation that many patients will affirm that their childhood was a happy time until analysis reveals that their parents were indifferent, insensitive, and sometimes cruel. They have blocked their early memories because they are too painful and too frightening to accept. But when childhood is lost to the mature consciousness, so also is the open and full-hearted love of the infant and the innocence of the child. Actually, neither the stages nor the memories are lost; they are sequestered and encapsulated.

The confusion of identity that results when a person's sexuality is neither accepted nor respected is illustrated in the following case. Jenny, a very bright woman in her thirties, and herself a therapist, consulted me because she found it very difficult to relate to people. She believed that they were not open and direct with her. On the other hand, she could not be open and direct with them, for she feared that any self-assertion, any statement of feeling, would provoke an attack. In self-defense she adopted a negative attitude—I don't want or need them—which was not true but served to protect her from a feared rejection or humiliation. She was split between her longing to be recognized and accepted and her denial of these feelings, which made her feel crazy at times. Her pain was so great that she would cry to herself for hours alone. When she cried in a group setting, it was painful to watch, because no one could reach her.

Who was Jenny? She didn't know because she was very confused. However, her body revealed the source of her confusion. She had a small head and face and a large, well-developed body.

Her face was twisted in an expression of pain, sadness, and bitterness. It was not an attractive-looking face. Surprisingly, her body was attractive: it was large, well shaped, and womanly. Her legs were strong and looked as if they could support her. She was an independent person both financially and psychologically but not emotionally. There were visible areas of tension in her body, notably around the shoulders and chest and about the pelvis.

The disharmony between Jenny's head and body can be interpreted as follows: Her head and face represented her ego, the part of her body that she presented to the world. The small size of her head and the tortured look of her face signified that her ego had been badly hurt and greatly damaged. The fullness, vitality and strength of the rest of her body indicated that she had been well nurtured as a very young child. The damage to her ego and the destruction of her sense of self had to have taken place at a later age, probably during the Oedipal period, when her ego was developing.

Jenny was the only girl in a family of seven children. In such a situation one could imagine that she was the focus of seven pairs of masculine eyes. Their interest in her as a female could have made her feel admired and desirable. Unfortunately, it didn't work out that way. She related an incident that shocked me. She said that on occasion her brothers surrounded her and urinated on her. She believed that her mother knew of this but made no effort to stop it or to discipline the boys. Her father was not at home much of the time and of no help to her. She described him as passive but said that she felt that he had warm feelings for her. These warm feelings for her and his acceptance of her as a sexual person allowed her to have positive sexual feelings. However, his sexual interest in her aroused the jealousy of her mother. Unfortunately for Jenny, he did not protect her against her mother's jealousy.

Her mother, on the other hand, terrified her. She could never do anything to please her mother, who constantly criticized her and often slapped her in the face. As we discussed her mother, Jenny realized that her mother had some insanity in her. She described a recent incident in which she, her mother, her brother, and his family were riding in a car in Switzerland. The mother made her brother stop the car, whereupon she took over the wheel and drove the car over Alpine roads at such speed that Jenny was sure the car would go out of control and they would all plunge to disaster. Yet this mother looked at Jenny as if she were the crazy one and called her that at times.

It is not surprising that Jenny herself thought she must be crazy. In a way she was, for she was confused about her reality and the reality about her. It is impossible for a very young child to see and recognize insanity in a mother unless the mother is hospitalized or the mother's insanity is acknowledged by the rest of the family. A young child takes the blame for her mother's behavior upon herself since her mother is the ground and reality of her being and to question that reality feels crazy. As a child, Jenny also sensed that her femininity aroused an excitement in her brothers, and yet they treated her with hostility and contempt. Their behavior could only be explained by assuming that they were acting out what they sensed was their mother's feeling toward the girl. At the same time they were taking out on Jenny their anger at their mother, of whom they, too, were afraid. Jenny was the scapegoat.

This mother could not accept Jenny's sexuality because she could not accept her own. If a mother regards her own sexuality as disgusting or dirty, she will see her daughter in that light. Most mothers unconsciously project the feelings they have about themselves on their daughters.

In the course of therapy, Jenny expressed a hatred for her mother that appalled her. Again and again, she cried out, "I hate you," with a vehemence that spoke of a murderous rage. Such an intense feeling can make a person feel crazy if it is not understood and accepted. To accept such a feeling, it needs to be expressed but not acted out, since it belongs to the past. The proper place for such an expression is in a therapy situation. As Jenny expressed her hatred of her mother in therapy, she became aware that her mother had hated her on a sexual level, though she had been able to love and accept her as a nonsexual infant. As Jenny's sexual nature developed and she responded initially to her brothers' interest in her, her mother began to see her as bad. The split in the mother created the split in the child.

Jenny was a sexual person but only from the shoulders down. She said that she liked men and enjoyed sex with them but found it very difficult to form a relationship. She was seriously split between her sexual desires, her fear of opening her heart, and her negative thinking. When this picture became clear in the course of therapy, Jenny felt the light of understanding and the warmth of recognition and acceptance. She remarked: "I believe I could be pretty. My face feels softer and less tense now." She added, "I would like to have a man." Healing the split in a patient's personality is the major task of therapy.

We have seen that as a result of the Oedipal experiences described above, childhood becomes encapsulated: that is, removed to some degree from consciousness. Another way of describing the situation is to say that the person loses touch with the child he was. At the same time, his heart becomes surrounded by a protective armoring that, in effect, locks it up in a cage (Fig. 9). No longer is it free to respond to the world outside. Growth will proceed through the next three stages, but the person will be estranged from his deepest and earliest feelings.

The effect is to split the unity of the personality. Instead of an integrated individual who is loving, joyful, adventurous, romantic, and responsible, the person has two antithetical centers of being, each with its own mode of being and acting.

Figure 10 illustrates this concept. One center exists around the heart and its associated feelings: love, playfulness, innocence, joy. It is the deep center in each individual. The second center,

Figure 9. The encapsulating of childhood experiences in the total personality. The impulse to reach out with love from the heart is restrained by the armor and can surface only tentatively.

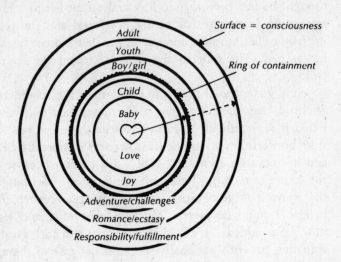

Figure 10. Splitting the unity into an ego (adult) center and a heart (infant/child) center. All impulses to reach out stem from the heart. Where a split exists, if the feeling of love is strong, the adult (ego) component is weak. Where the ego (adult) feeling is strong, the feeling of love is weak.

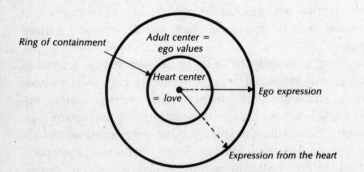

Figure 11. The unified personality. There is free and full communication between all aspects of the personality.

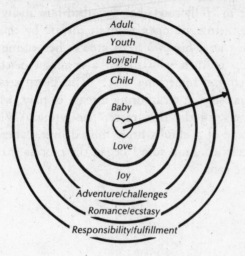

dominated by the ego, is at the surface, where contact with the world is made. Its associated feelings are the desire for recognition and status, the drive to achieve and succeed, and the urge for self-expression. In a healthy person, heart feelings and ego drives do not conflict. The drive to achieve is the mature extension of the child's pleasure in play, and the urge for self-expression is related to the child's joy in bodily movement and creative activity. This integrated personality is shown in figure 11.

In the split individual, the reaching out for love has an infantile quality that is manifested in the desire to be taken care of, to be held and protected, to be nurtured. The reaching out stems from emptiness, not fullness. However, when the person reaches out from his second or ego center, he comes across as superindependent, superaggressive, and seemingly in command of himself. This attitude covers and hides the needy and vulnerable child within by creating a facade that is its exact opposite.

Denying one's vulnerability doesn't eliminate it; it simply

transfers it from the surface to the center, from the ego to the heart, which becomes susceptible to a heart attack. Clancy Sigal, a writer in Hollywood, has described how many successful men leave themselves open to heart disease by this denial. Sigal found that after his own heart attack, he became a member of a group of men who shared a common defect and a common search for something lost. "The heart attack may become the first step in recapturing a sense of play, whose loss led to the attack in the first place," he wrote. "When that special landscape of a child's heart misted over, when I grew tough and 'realistic,' I am sure I began the process that landed me in intensive care."[3]

CHAPTER 4

The Loss of Love and the Loss of Hope: "I Can't Live Without You"

In chapter 1 we examined the positive effects that love has on the heart. Love causes the heart to beat faster and stronger, sending more blood to the surface of the body, brightening the eyes, and charging the erogenous areas. In love a person reaches out for closeness and contact in anticipation of pleasure. If nothing disturbs the relationship with the love object, such an impulse is full and free, and the person feels lighthearted and gay. When contact is established, there is a feeling of pleasure, contentment, and peace. The excitement subsides, the heart quiets down, one feels filled with a sense of well-being. But what happens when a move to establish contact with another meets with rejection, when the loved person is unavailable or even lost? Instead of pleasure, one feels pain; instead of fulfillment, one feels emptiness; instead of the peace and contentment that follows the release of excitement, one feels tense and distraught.

Many of us have experienced at some time or other the pain

that accompanies the loss of love. A young woman whose mother was dying placed her hand over her heart and said, "It hurts so much. I feel my heart will break." This pain is a real physical sensation located in the region of the heart. What causes it?

When a person experiences a loss of love, the blood that had been sent to the surface of the body in anticipation of closeness (even the thought of contact with or closeness to the loved person can excite the heart and send the blood to the surface) is suddenly withdrawn to the interior, to the heart itself. The heart is now engorged with more blood than it can easily expel. The pressure builds, and the heart feels as if it would burst. At the same time, the chest muscles contract. Actually, the whole body goes into a state of contraction as a reaction to the loss of love. This is the opposite of the state of expansion that love produces.

In most cases, the person does burst—into sobs or occasionally into screams. Such a reaction often occurs when a loved one dies. The screaming and crying are so intense that the person seems to be crying as if his heart were broken. What breaks down is the rigidity that develops in the wake of a loss. One can clearly see this process of breaking down when a baby begins to cry following some hurt or disappointment. His first reaction to hurt is to stiffen. An adult can maintain such a state, but an infant cannot. A few moments after the shock, the baby's jaw begins to quiver, which leads immediately to crying. Crying in a baby is a convulsive reaction that embraces the whole body and gives rise to loud sounds of distress as air in the lungs is expelled.

Crying is the most basic form of release the human organism has available to discharge the tension resulting from pain. A baby's crying is also a call for help, a call for his mother and therefore a reaction to the loss of love. Sobbing, or continuous crying, is unique to the human species. The cries of other mammals take the form of single sounds. Shedding tears is also limited to human beings. These special responses suggest that people can experience not only a greater degree of sorrow than other mammals but also more intense feelings of love, partly because the human brain is better able to perceive subtle states of feeling and sensation but largely because the human body is more excitable. The increased excitability of the human animal is most obvious in its sexuality. Whereas almost all other mammals are limited in their sexual responsiveness to specific rut periods, the adult human's sexual responsiveness is largely independent of the reproductive cycle. With the increased frequency of sexual desire, the urge for closeness and intimacy is more pressing, producing heightened feelings of love and, when loss occurs, of sorrow.

To cope with loss, nature, fortunately, has provided a strong release mechanism in sobbing. While tears streaming down the face are also an expression of sadness, that expression does not provide the bodily relief that sobbing does. The flow of tears serves to release tension in the eyes, which is evident in the fact that most people's eyes are softer and brighter after a good cry. But body rigidity, especially the armoring in the chest produced by the pain of the loss of love, can only be released by sobbing.

In a baby, the tension resulting from the experience of hurt or pain is acute and can be quickly released. But in many adults the tension is chronic, and the release of that tension through crying is not easy. This is especially true of men, some of whom find it almost impossible to cry. It may take considerable therapy to soften an individual to the point where he can react emotionally to the loss of love. Jack had been in therapy for a number of years before he could cry. Following a conflict in which his girlfriend told him that she wasn't ready to live with him, he described his reaction as follows:

> I just felt my heart break. I didn't say anything. I went and cried very deeply that night. My chest ached all week. And I felt—this is it, it's finished. It was the same feeling that I had

when my first girlfriend and I broke up. I kept to myself that week, but I also had the very strong feeling that I wanted someone to share my life and my love. We met again at the end of the week, and again she announced her independence. My pain came back. My chest had been hurting all week. It was painful. I felt so tired. I said, "I just can't stand this," and I started to cry. I think I cried more deeply than I can ever remember crying before. I bawled and bawled and bawled with her there, which I believe was important. As I cried, I felt my heart break. I really hurt in my heart. I'll be damned! When I was done, my chest felt clear. It didn't hurt anymore. I felt freer and free with Helen.

Before, I always felt that pain was being inflicted on me. Now I felt it as *my* heartbreak. Owning up, I was able to clean it out. You know, I try to be the big shot, but I see how very vulnerable I am to the feeling of abandonment because of this heartbreak in me. I'm vulnerable to sexual rejection.

The pain of a cut finger is strictly limited to the area of injury. But emotional pain, unlike a purely physical injury, involves the whole body. People speak of a weight on the chest, difficulty in breathing, and a feeling of constriction in addition to the specific pain in the heart itself. But not everyone experiences a loss of love with the same intensity. Many people have developed such powerful defenses against emotional hurts and pains that the breakup of a love relationship leaves them cold, depressed, or without feeling. These are individuals who do not feel the joy of love, either.

The heartbreak that made Jack feel vulnerable to rejection stemmed from experiences in early childhood. After another crisis with his girlfriend, Jack himself made the connection to the loss of his mother's breast:

I felt very keenly the loss of physical contact with my girlfriend, of touching and holding her, of the excitement of erotic contact. The feeling of that loss is a physical memory—the loss of all nurturing, life-giving, comforting, and fulfilling skin contact with my mother. It was a feeling of coldness and emptiness. As my crying deepened, I began to gasp for air, and I could sense the panic this feeling of loss evoked.

When the loss of love occurs in childhood, it leaves the individual with a persistent underlying panic. But just as the pain of heartbreak is repressed, the feeling of panic is suppressed and rises to consciousness only when he attempts to breathe deeply and finds that he cannot get enough air. Such a reaction occurs whenever a person feels trapped in a life-threatening situation. He will make every possible effort to escape, but if panic seizes him, his efforts will be chaotic, and therefore futile. When people feel trapped by a fire, they rush blindly to the nearest exit and end up blocking the exit so that escape is impossible. There are often other escape routes, but panic precludes the exercise of any rational judgment. We all know that clear thinking is imperative in a situation of danger, but such thinking requires an adequate supply of oxygen to the brain. If the breath is held, as it is in a state of fear, the oxygen supply to the brain drops precipitously, and clear thinking becomes impossible.

All fear affects the breathing. Our instinctive reaction is to suck in our breath, raise our shoulders, and open our eyes wide. This reaction, known as the startle reaction, can be observed in infants when they are frightened by a loud noise or by the threat of falling when support is suddenly withdrawn. Not all adults panic under the same conditions. The more secure a person is, the more his breathing remains relatively free and unconstricted, and the less likely he is to panic. The inner sense of security stems from early experiences of feeling loved and accepted. In contrast, the person who suffered a lack of acceptance lacks this sense of security.

An important question to ask is why a loss of love in childhood makes a person feel insecure all his life despite the fact that he may have a loving relationship with a wife or partner. The answer is that the insecurity is structured in his body on an unconscious level. Though he may have some general awareness of being insecure, he does not connect his insecurity to his tight throat or his inflated chest. Nor does he really feel the extent to which he holds himself up by his shoulders instead of allowing his legs and feet to support him.

Since our legs and feet are our functional roots, connecting us to the ground when we stand or move, it is easy to see why such a person lacks a sense of security. His legs may look strong, but if they are tight and rigid, sensation in them will be diminished, and it will be difficult for him to feel a sense of support. Such rigidity must be seen as a defense against the fear of falling. This fear first arises when an infant feels he lacks support. As an adult, he still feels unconsciously that if he fell, not only would nobody be there to pick him up, but the very ground might fall away beneath him.

To an infant, his mother is the actual ground. If her support is insufficient, the child will develop the sense that he cannot count on anyone but himself and that he must hold himself up by his own conscious effort. Eventually that effort becomes unconscious. As long as the child—and later, the adult—holds himself up by tensing his shoulders and by tightening his legs, he will feel insecure in life.

Any loss of love or security, any situation of fear or danger, can aggravate this underlying insecurity, evoking a strong feeling of panic. Many women suffer from agoraphobia, a fear of being alone in an open space. *Agora* is the Greek word for marketplace, and beneath such a reaction is the fear of being separated from one's mother in a crowded place. That leaving the house evokes the same reaction in a grown woman is related to an unconscious fear of separation or abandonment. The problem is difficult to treat because agoraphobics are rarely aware that their panic stems from early experiences with their mothers.

Migraine is another symptom that can be related to the loss of love and the fear of abandonment. One of my patients came in for treatment precisely because she suffered from such severe migraines that she was incapacitated at times. Mary was an attractive young woman in her late twenties with a bright, lively manner and a ready smile, except when her face became twisted under the excruciating pain of a severe attack. Getting Mary to cry deeply relieved the headache; if done early enough, sometimes it aborted the attack. When she cried, some of the tension seemed to go out of her body, especially around her eyes and head. Screaming was even more effective in diminishing the pain. Still, for all her pain, it wasn't easy for Mary to break down and sob. It was part of her personality structure to be in control, to be bright and cheerful, and to be effective in the world. However, since her control was based on denial, she couldn't handle her feelings, especially the sexual ones, when they arose, and so she was in constant conflict. She would often get a headache just before going out on a date and would have to cancel it, though this did not stop the headache. She also took antimigraine medication constantly, though it was not fully effective. In therapy she came to understand the conflicts in her personality that created the tension behind her headaches.

Mary came from an Irish Catholic family in which sex and sexual matters were covered up and regarded as sinful. She was very much attached to her father, and his death, when she was ten years old, came as a great shock. However, she did not break down and cry. Since her father died in a hospital, her mother, thinking to spare her, did not tell Mary of his death immediately, and Mary seized on this delay to deny that he was irretrievably gone. Instead, she imagined him to be in heaven watching her all the time, and she believed that if she were a good girl (which meant not to be sexual), he would somehow come back to her. As an adult, Mary no longer believed that he would come back, but in the course of therapy it became clear that on an unconscious level she had not fully accepted the fact of his death. At issue was her inability to react emotionally. Why?

Mary had looked to her father as a protector against her

mother, whom she saw as hostile and as a competitor for her father's affections. His loss left her in an intolerable state of vulnerability and defenselessness. To compensate, she envisioned him in heaven, where she could still think of him as her protector. In reality, the pain of his loss was too great for her to bear and, therefore, to acknowledge. As she put it some time later, "I couldn't bear it. I would have died if I had admitted he was dead." Whether Mary would have died or not is immaterial; she simply could not act against such a strong feeling.

The denial of her father's loss transferred the pain to her head. The mechanism for this transfer hinged upon Mary's attempts to deny and control her sexuality. In her unconscious mind, Mary blamed the loss of her father on her sexual feelings toward him. She was a bad girl, and his loss was her punishment. If she were not sexual, she might still be connected to her father and, thus, be spared the heartbreak of his loss. This control of sexual feeling was accomplished by diverting the blood from the genitals to the head, resulting in the engorgement and pulsing of the arteries in the brain. Support for this view of the psychopathology of migraine was given by the great reduction in the frequency and intensity of Mary's headaches as her sexual guilt and the denial of her loss were worked through in therapy.[1] But Mary could only accept her loss if she could release its pain by deeply mourning her father's death through sobbing and crying.

The importance of crying to release the tension and relieve the pain of heartbreak cannot be overstressed. The loss of a loved person must be mourned if one is to resume a normal life after the loss. Psychologists since Freud have known that the failure to mourn an important loss sets up the individual for depression or melancholia.[2] All depressive reactions have their roots in a loss of love that has not been properly mourned.[3] Depression subsequently develops out of the illusion that the lost love can be regained by "good" behavior.

To deny the death of a loved parent is not that common,

because it introduces an element of unreality into the child's life that disturbs its relationship to other people. It occurs when the attachment to that parent is so powerful that the loss cannot be accepted. On the other hand, to deny the loss of love is quite common. Few people are willing to admit that they were unloved as children. Even patients in therapy have considerable difficulty accepting this possibility. Generally, it is only after they have experienced the pain of their heartbreak that they are willing to recognize that one or both parents had been considerably hostile toward them. If they describe acts of insensitivity or cruelty on the part of a parent, they justify such behavior by blaming themselves or excuse it by sympathizing with the parent's pain and suffering. Often the more abused a child has been, the less willing or able he is to see that abuse as an expression of hatred. For a child to accept the fact of parental hatred is to question the order of nature. And yet the reality, as we adults see it, is that parents are ambivalent about their children. On the one hand, they wish the best for them; on the other, however, they resent their demands. They are also envious of the child, who seems to have more than they did when they were children.

Such ambivalence is evident in the degree to which parental love is conditioned upon a child's achievements and accomplishments. In our culture, where success has become the most important "virtue," many parents see their children's accomplishments as a mark of their own superiority. Too often their egos are involved in their children's status and performance in and out of school. But a love conditioned upon performance is not love at all. True love surrounds a person with warmth and affection for who he is and not what he does. "Mother will love you if you eat all your cereal" is not a statement of love but of rejection. The same goes for statements like "You are so dirty. How can anyone love you?" A child is born a little animal, and if his mother's love is conditioned upon his being trained for civilized living, his basic nature is rejected. All children have to adapt to social living, but this process does not require threats and punishments. Just as children learn to speak spontaneously and naturally, they also learn in time how to be well behaved and courteous. True, they are not always quiet and still, which upsets those parents unable to stand the liveliness of their children.

Psychologists are aware that today's children are under enormous pressure to grow up quickly, a fact that they attribute to the competitive nature of our culture. But another reason to pressure children to grow up is to free harried parents from the stress of having to devote their time and energy to their needs. How many mothers find fulfillment in nursing their babies? How many fathers have the time, the patience, and the energy to rock a baby to sleep? The initial heartbreak occurs when the baby senses that his desires and needs are secondary and that no matter how much he cries, he will not get the attention and caring he wants.

Children soon learn that by being there emotionally for their parents, they gain some measure of approval and affection. "I had to be a mother to my mother" is a remark often heard in therapy. Children are sensitive to their parents' suffering and make every effort to alleviate it. As one patient said, "I couldn't cry because I couldn't burden my mother with my sadness. She had so much sadness of her own to cope with." The child suppresses his own longing and tries to be the kind of person who can make the parent happy. At first, this means being good and obedient, an attitude reinforced in school. It is not difficult to see the progression from pleasing one's parents to performing in school to achieving success in one's career. This commitment to pleasing others can have no other basis than the hope and belief that it will earn the person love and overcome the heartbreak he experienced earlier in life.

However, this behavior no more works for the adult than it did for the child. Of course, the adult is unaware that he seeks to earn love by his actions, since he has suppressed his longing for love. But this longing breaks through from time to time, together with the feeling of being trapped in a hopeless situation. Both feelings, longing and hopelessness, threaten to undermine the person's defense against the feeling of heartbreak and open the gates to a flood of sadness in which he fears he may drown. Still, the impulse to break out and to find love, no matter how painful, will inevitably arise, and with it a feeling of panic at the prospect of being abandoned again. (The relationship of heart attack to the breakthrough of panic will be explored in a subsequent chapter.)

The ambivalence of parents toward their children is not only manifested in a lukewarm attitude or in a lack of sufficient nurturing. Some parents feel downright hostile toward their offspring. The effect of such hatred on a child is different from the effect of parental narcissism, as described above. It is one thing to be panicked at the prospect of abandonment and quite another to be terrified by a parent's hostility. Child abuse, a well-known phenomenon today, may involve physical beatings that go so far as to endanger or even to destroy the life of a child, or it may involve a more psychological form of warfare. I recall a dinner with a family at which the mother forbade her young son to touch his favorite meat dish until he had eaten all the vegetables on his plate. The boy, who for some reason had an aversion to vegetables, struggled with his mother's harsh directive but couldn't quite swallow it. I felt sorry for him and interceded on his behalf with his mother. I'll not forget the look of hatred she turned on me for my seemingly unjustified interference. Her child turned out to have serious emotional problems.

On another occasion, I was consulted by a mother with her daughter, who also had some serious problems. As the girl talked to me, I happened to glance at her mother and found her looking at the girl with black, hate-filled eyes. Yet as we talked, she denied any hostile feelings toward the girl. She was obviously unaware of her inner feelings, but I am sure her daughter had seen and been terrified by this black look many times.

Terror is a different kind of fear than panic. When a predator threatens a herd of animals, they stampede, running wildly to escape. But once a predator captures his prey, the animal generally is so terrified that it cannot make a conscious effort to escape. Terror not only paralyzes the animal but numbs it, thereby decreasing the pain of its death agony.

Children who are terrified by their parents lose the ability to fight back and can only submit helplessly to the situation. They cease to feel anything because all spontaneous movement toward or away from the parent stops. Such a child may become slavishly attached to the hateful parent, but that attachment stems from fear, not love. The effect of terror on the body is also different from the effect of panic. Instead of rigidity, there is a tendency toward flaccidity; instead of an inflated chest, one sees a deflated chest; and instead of the aggressivity associated with Type A behavior, one finds a great deal of passivity in the personality. Having said this, I would caution the reader against classifying individuals into types, since few people grow up experiencing terror or panic exclusively. On one occasion a child may panic when his crying fails to bring his mother; on another he may become terrified when his crying evokes a hostile reaction from his father. Parental behavior is rarely consistent, varying as it does with the mood of the parent. Even the most hateful parent has positive feelings for his child now and then.

Rarely does the loving connection between a parent and child rupture completely. Both minor and major breaks can occur and last for different lengths of time. Each break may cause some anguish to a child, but the intensity of that anguish will vary from one family to another and from one child to another in the same family. Similarly, a child will not encounter a fixed amount of hostility or hatred from a parent. Generally hostility flares from time to time. However, in other cases the child may be aware of a persistent hostility that rarely lifts.

Since most people have a short memory for the pain they experienced as children, it is the rare patient who can describe his childhood accurately. In most cases, patients deny the negative aspects or gloss them over, but the experiences of childhood are structured in the body all the same. The inflated, armored chest is a defense against present panic and past heartbreak. The degree of rigidity reveals the severity of the early trauma. The deflated or collapsed chest denotes the effect of terror on the heart, a crushing blow against which no defense is possible. In such cases the body shows an absence of rigidity.

We saw in chapter 3 that the loss of love splits the unity of the personality, creating two centers, the ego center and the heart center. The latter is cut off from the conscious sense of self. The ego is weakened in the process, but it remains strong enough to maintain a coherent sense of self despite the existence of serious internal conflicts. Such an individual is determined to avoid the possibility of heartbreak by gaining love through service, hard work, and achievement or through the allure of power and success. The overall rigidity of his body serves to create a superficial unity in his personality. This unity is lacking in the schizoid individual, who has been crushed. In the process, his spirit is broken but not his heart, leaving him less vulnerable than the rigid individual to heart disease. His heart is also more open to love, but the love he seeks tends to be infantile or childish. At the same time, he is less focused on achievement.

Figures 12a and 12b are useful in illustrating the different dynamics of these personality structures. Figure 12a represents the rigid structure (narcissistic personality), which is associated with underlying panic. As the diagram demonstrates, the ego center (shaded area) dominates the personality, while the heart center is closed off. The double line surrounding the whole indicates that personality boundaries are well defined and defended. A relatively strong charge exists at the surface of the body, ensuring good and stable contact with the external world. On the other hand, contact with the heart and its feelings is reduced.

Figure 12a. The rigid or narcissistic personality

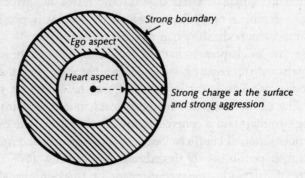

Figure 12b. The oral or schizoid personality

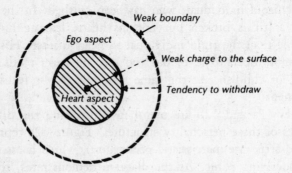

Fig. 12b represents the oral or schizoid personality structure, which is associated with underlying terror. In this structure, the opposite condition exists—namely, a weak ego with strong heart feelings. The shaded center denotes the dominance of the heart. Because of a reduced surface charge, the ego boundary of the schizoid structure is weak and undefended, with the result that the person is oversensitive, easily hurt, and likelier to withdraw than to fight in response to insults or traumas.

Tony was a person who showed some features of both conditions, although unconscious panic predominated. His complaint—depression and a lack of feeling—is common enough these days. According to Tony, life offered him no excitement; he admitted that he could lie in bed all day, watching television. Almost all movement for him required some action of his will, since he had immobilized his body to such an extent that no spontaneous movement or emotion could occur. He was well built and muscular, but an unusual degree of tension in his voluntary muscles had rigidified his body. Because his shoulders were raised and fixed, he had great difficulty extending his arms over his head. His chest was highly overinflated; consequently, his breathing was very limited. Of course, he couldn't cry, although the expression on his face when he relaxed was sad and unhappy.

Tony was an only child. He had almost no memories of his childhood and could recall very few instances when his parents had expressed any affection for him. Since his mother used to play cards every day with her friends, when he came home from school there was never anyone to greet him. His father had taken him occasionally to ball games but had also beat him whenever he disobeyed or caused any trouble. Tony could not recall the beatings in much detail except to say that he used to hide under the bed from his father and to put books in his pants so that the spankings would hurt less. He often mentioned the size of his father's hands, as if to say that they had frightened him, but he expressed no fear or any other feeling in his accounts. He was a lonely child with almost no friends or companions. As an adolescent, he stole money from his father to take out his friends so that he would not be so alone.

It was possible to detect signs of Tony's relationship to his parents in his body. In reaction to the hostility of his father, he had stiffened as if to say, "You're not going to break me. I won't cry no matter how much you hit me." And he hadn't cried when his father beat him. In response to the indifference and withdrawal of his mother, he had hardened his heart as if to say, "I don't need you. I don't need anybody. I don't care if nobody loves me." But Tony was not hard-hearted. In fact, he had a very soft heart and was sensitive to the pain and suffering of his children and friends—for he, too, had suffered greatly. The hardness was on the surface, an armoring to protect himself from the coldness and hostility of the world and the suffering within. But he was also numbed and paralyzed by the terror he felt for his father, which increased his difficulty in opening up and reaching out for love.

When Tony did an exercise in deep breathing, he didn't break down as others had. Nor did he panic or feel much pain. He did feel uncomfortable, and his shoulders hurt enough that he couldn't stay long with the exercise. As a result, his breathing didn't deepen significantly, and no emotion was aroused. Clearly, Tony was afraid to let go. Fortunately, he was aware of holding on too tightly, especially as it manifested itself in the spasticity of his muscles, and he recognized it as a form of resistance. Part of him felt determined not to break down in therapy any more than he had as a child when his father hit him. Knowing this made it possible for him to stay with the therapy, despite very slow progress. The process of helping Tony learn to cry was a long one, but the alternative was the living death of no feeling. The latter was so distressing that on a number of occasions Tony exclaimed, "I wish I was dead."

The rigidity and tension in Tony's chest marked him as a candidate for a heart attack. He was subject to an enormous amount of physical stress, stemming from the tension in the muscles of his body. If stress were the sole factor determining a heart attack, Tony would have had little chance to avoid one, but he had a way of minimizing stress that had saved him so far. He did not push or drive himself. As he said, he could lie in bed all day. His underlying hopelessness prevented him from trying to achieve and to gain love. Despite his indifference to success, he had built a very successful business, thanks to his supersharp intelligence and his ability to let others work for him. The extreme rigidity and numbness of his body left his mind free to function objectively in the world. Unable to feel and to act, Tony resorted to thinking. He lived in his head, doing a crossword puzzle every day. Fortunately, he was intelligent enough to know that he needed to change and that it could only be done by making his body become more alive. He succeeded with the help of the body work that is part of bioenergetic therapy.

After a number of years in therapy, Tony had a short, unusual dream. "I dreamt I was going to die of cancer in a week," he recounted. "Very calmly, I made my plans to dispose of my property." One week after this dream, Tony fell in love. The connection is clear to me. Tony had expressed the wish to die several times, but he had never accepted it. He was a survivor, and he didn't need love or anybody. He believed that his survival depended on his denial of his feelings, but through the dream he realized that denial was the road to death. To live is to love. To deny the desire for love is a living death that will inevitably end in a fatal illness. In the dream, Tony recognized that he would die if he didn't open himself to love.

Was Tony unique in equating survival with not loving, not caring? His was an extreme position, but the fear of love is widespread despite the fact that few would deny love's importance. Since this fear is at the root of the predisposition to heart disease, we will examine it in some detail in the next chapter.

CHAPTER 5

The Fear of Love

I have described the split in the personality between the child and the adult, between the feelings of the heart and the drives of the ego. Such a split characterizes the rigid individual, who identifies primarily with the ego and with the adult person he has become. As we have seen, rigidity is a defense against the pain of early heartbreak and the possibility that the heart might be broken again. Associated with it is an unconscious fear of abandonment, which amounts to a fear of love itself. If we don't love, we risk no loss of love, and we cannot be abandoned. But we are trapped behind our own defenses, which by their very existence ensures that our worst fears are justified.

The defense of the rigid individual is built into his ego structure. To surrender it entails a regression from adult to child and an apparent loss of the self-esteem that he has worked so hard to achieve. One patient described this dilemma very clearly. She was a thirty-year-old divorced woman who had been in an unsatisfying relationship with a man for two years, during which time she complained about his lack of serious interest in her. One day, she reported, he declared that he was prepared to make a serious commitment. "I had stopped complaining and was feeling some love for him when he said he wanted more, to be closer," she said. "I became frightened and began to sob. If I let myself go, I would get hurt. If he left me, I would be devastated. If he didn't leave me, I would merge with him and lose my identity. I would be nobody."

How could she feel herself to be nobody if she surrendered to love? All our songs and poems tell us that surrendering to love ennobles rather than diminishes us. We can understand this apparent contradiction only if we realize that while the feeling of being in love is a positive and exciting state, the prospect of falling in love may be frightening to some people because it involves a surrender of ego control. To the extent that this patient's sense of self depended on her ego, she would feel like nobody if she abandoned that position. On the other hand, if her sense of self had been based on the feelings in her body, the surrender of ego control would have enhanced her sense of self, and she would have felt herself to be truly somebody. Individuals who have cut off bodily feeling as a defense against the pain of heartbreak base their identity on their ability to control feeling. This control gives them a sense of power that substitutes for a true sense of self. Power creates the illusion that they are somebody. It is, as we shall see in this chapter, the recourse of people who are afraid to love.

The idea that love entails a merger of two people is true only of the symbiotic relationship of an infant and his mother. As the infant grows and becomes more independent, the relationship changes. Independence means that the child is somebody in his own right. While full independence is not established until maturity, the child's sense of being somebody starts quite early and is fairly well established by six years of age. The process depends, however, on the nurturing, support, and love of the child's parents. The child is handicapped or even blocked by a lack or a loss of love. In this situation, normal development does not occur, and the child remains emotionally fixated at an early level despite the fact that he continues to grow and eventually reaches sexual maturity. On a deep level—that is, in his heart—such a person remains a child who has not fully separated from his mother to become a viable somebody. On the surface, he appears to be mature and independent, but these traits are not grounded in a fullness of being or rooted in the security of love. To surrender this position threatens to return him to the emotional state of infancy and childhood, a frightening prospect indeed to someone who grew up feeling helpless, dependent, and lacking a secure sense of self.

Since such a person needs to love but is afraid to open himself fully to love, he works out arrangements with his partners in which they use each other. They may well feel some affection for each other, but the arrangement serves primarily to mask the fear of surrender. These arrangements are not conscious; they duplicate the arrangement a person had with his mother or father. As long as the arrangement works, it allays the fear of abandonment, but it is not deeply satisfying, for it cannot substitute for love.

We need only to scratch the surface of most relationships to find the arrangement beneath. Most often, it goes something like this: If you are there for me in my need, I'll be there for you in yours. One patient expressed this idea succinctly when he said about his marriage, "I play father to her little girl, and she plays mother to my little boy." Such an arrangement may sound workable, but in fact this patient harbored tremendous hostility toward his mother for keeping him a little boy, hostility that he transferred to his wife. He had not recognized that his marriage was held together by an arrangement until it came apart at the seams. He resented being treated like a little boy by a woman who was herself emotionally immature. Still, he could not leave his wife because the knowledge that she needed him gave him some sense of security. In general, people hedge their relationships in this fashion out of a fear of abandonment. Only by confronting the underlying panic is it possible to deal with the problem.

Paul, a forty-year-old doctor, found out as much during one therapy session. "There is a tension in my chest," he told me. "Something in there wants to come out." Suddenly it struck him then that the feeling in his chest was one of sadness. "I'm afraid of my sadness," he admitted. "I sense how lonely I've been. I don't dare open my heart." As the feeling of sadness deepened, he exclaimed, "How could you do this to me? You're breaking my heart." Paul spoke in the present tense because he was reliving the experience of heartbreak. As we talked about the feeling in his chest, he remarked, "There's nothing in there, no feeling. It feels empty. I don't feel my heart." I interpreted his statement to mean that he didn't feel the love in his heart. To reach the love that he had blocked off at an early age to protect himself, Paul had to regress to the stage of infancy. Lying on the couch, he reached out softly with his lips like an infant wanting to suck. As he did so, he felt the longing he had suppressed for his mother and began to cry. "I want you," he said, adding, "I get scared."

Paul's childhood is similar to that of others I have presented. When his father died, Paul became the little man of the house. His mother was seductive with him, inviting an intimate relationship, but when he expressed any sexual interest in her, she humiliated and controlled him. This relationship was perverted because Paul invariably had to put his mother's wishes and needs before his own. Out of guilt for his sexual feelings and fearful that he might be abandoned, he promised to be a good boy.

In therapy, Paul was able to acknowledge his sadness and discuss his relationship with his mother. "I'm feeling for the first time what I felt as a kid," he remarked. "Poor little kid. It makes me mad." And then he got out some of his anger by hitting the bed.

This incident from Paul's therapy was just one of the several dramatic episodes that allowed him to gain insight into his personality. Before entering therapy, he had been unaware that he was not a loving person, since he had had plenty of relationships with women to whom he felt attached. However, those relationships duplicated his relationship to his mother, to whom he was still attached. He took care of them, he was "there" for them, and, in return, they were "there" for him in a sexual way. These relationships were based not on passion or deep feeling but on need. Paul needed his lovers sexually, and they needed his interest and support. Some people use this kind of interdependency as a basis for marriage, but Paul was looking for something deeper and richer—for love. As a result, he never married. Try as he might, he couldn't find love, essentially because he wasn't open to it.

Paul saw himself as a man who could and would take care of a woman. It gave him a sense of power and superiority that compensated for his inner feeling of being a "poor little kid." As a poor little kid, he had felt helpless and powerless against the seduction and threats of his mother. However, compensating mechanisms only change the appearance of reality; on a sexual level, Paul was still the poor little kid whose mother had castrated psychologically. That castration was apparent in his inability to make his pitch for a woman on the basis of his sexual appeal rather than on his ability to serve her. The compensating role that he played did serve some purpose: It supported his erective potency by decreasing his fear of humiliation and rejection. Unfortunately, it also operated to reduce his orgasmic potency.

Such arrangements are based on what the parties believe are their needs. A woman, for example, may need to be admired for her cuteness, her brightness, and her flirtatious sexuality, just as she had as a little girl. But these qualities are more admirable in a child than in a woman. Yet many men do admire these qualities in women—they appeal not only to the little boy in them but to their need to feel manly and superior. This dovetailing of personalities might seem to be an ideal arrangement, but in practice it never works, because it does not fulfill either partner's true needs. A man may be excited by a woman who plays the role of a seductive little girl, but her lack of emotional maturity, especially on a sexual level, will eventually leave him dissatisfied. He will resent her dependence on him just as she will resent his superior pose, especially when he reveals the extent to which he needs her reassurance and support. After all, if there's a little boy in him, how can he take care of her? Sooner or later, what seemed like such a perfect love affair will disintegrate into recriminations and hostility.

To feel needed in a relationship may make us feel powerful and more secure, but that security is illusory, since power and love are opposite and antagonistic values. Power never really gains us love, especially power based on money or sex appeal. Power operates only to enhance the self-image, making us more ego conscious; love demands a surrender of the ego, while enhancing our bodily selves. We can't control another and claim to love him or her. By the same logic, we can't claim to be in love and to be in total control of ourselves. Self-control is an important element only in relationships where power is a factor. Unfortunately, parents commonly use power—in the form of punishment—in relation to their children.

Where punishment is concerned, it does not matter whether it is applied to criminals or to children; in either case, it is an exercise of power. Though it may be justified as a way to correct behavior, its real intent is to let the other person know who is boss. It can promote discipline, but it can just as easily foment rebellion. Its use with children is highly questionable. In the first place, they are innocent of evil intent; in the second, they look to parents as protectors, not as punishers. A small child experiences the act of physical punishment as a betrayal of his love and trust. How could he not! Of course, he is told that it is for his own good. Eventually, he may even come to believe that. If he does, he betrays himself by turning against his own feelings. Dog trainers avoid punishment when training a dog because they know there are better ways to accomplish their goals. Since dogs are eager to please, rewarding their good behavior is far more effective. As every trainer knows, training a dog requires patience—something many parents have in short supply in relation to their own children.

Since children lack any real power against their parents, they must submit when power is used against them. This submission is only on the surface, however. Inwardly, they develop a hard core of resistance. Most commonly, they will not cry when they are beaten or hurt. As we have seen, men who were beaten by their fathers as children find it very difficult to cry regardless of how much they are hurt. When this is discussed in therapy, they explain it as a form of defense. "I won't give him the satisfaction of seeing that he got to me," they say, as if their fathers were in the room. This defense becomes structured in the body as rigidity and is generalized to others. "No one is going to get to me" becomes their motto.

Some adults keep all their feelings from reaching the surface in response to abuses they suffered as children. A young woman whose facial expression was strongly masked explained it by saying, "My mother was always watching me, always studying my face. She seemed to take a perverse pleasure in knowing everything I felt. I had to hide my feelings from her." Not showing one's feelings may give one a sense of power in relationships, but at the same time it undermines the possibility of trust. In this way, self-control, which seems such an admirable quality, represents a fear of love.

Most relationships between men and women start with some feelings of love for each other, and most are wrecked by the power struggles that develop as the relationship becomes more intimate. It is said that familiarity breeds contempt. When a couple stops dating and starts living together, they are exposed to each other's weaknesses and faults, which they may pick on to gain a position of superiority. But criticism leads to defensiveness and breeds a critical attitude in return. As this happens, the excitement that brought them together in the first place diminishes, but they may stay together as a matter of convenience. However, such an arrangement leads to resentments. They find themselves trapped in a situation reminiscent in many ways of their childhood. They may get out of the relationship, struggle with it, or resign themselves to the loss of their hope for love and joy. But resignation can lead to cancer, while struggle often ends in a heart attack. Still, getting out is not the solution, since a second relationship often turns out to be no better than the first. To get out of this trap, the couple must deal with their fear of love.

On the deepest level, the fear of love is identical to fear of the opposite sex. Unconsciously, all men identify women with their mothers, just as women identify men with their fathers. This identification is natural. If our opposite-sex parent had been kind, loving, and strong, we would all have little difficulty with our mates. Unfortunately, this is rarely the case. Most people recall their relationship with that parent as one of conflict. Their experience was of being used, and their expectation was of being betrayed and hurt. Survival demanded a *modus vivendi*, an arrangement whereby we can live with some security by denying many of the negative aspects of these relationships and suppressing most of our negative feelings. But suppression only pushes these feelings below the level of consciousness; they remain operative in the personality in subtle and insidious ways.

Peter, like Tony in the previous chapter, came for therapy because he was depressed. He enjoyed neither his work nor his home life, and was in constant conflict with his wife, who accused him of being closed off to her and of withholding sex. He admitted that he was not excited by her and that he couldn't respond sexually when she approached him for intimacy. He also complained that she didn't accept him and made him feel guilty for his lack of interest. Peter found fault with her, as well: She was overweight, a sloppy housekeeper, and took too little responsibility for herself. Peter felt miserable, but when I suggested that he might leave the marriage, he resisted the idea. He had affectionate feelings for his wife, he said, and at times they got along. Besides, he didn't want to be alone. He realized that he was closed off and that he would have difficulty making any relationship with a woman work well. Being closed off also interfered with his relationships at work. Peter admitted he felt trapped, which added to his depression, but to get him out of it was no easy task; all the entangling forces in his personality stemming from his childhood had to be understood and released.

Peter was the youngest of three boys. When he was five, his parents separated, and the boys remained with their mother. Although Peter saw his father from time to time, he felt no real closeness to him. His mother disparaged his father constantly, which kept the boy alienated from him. His two brothers were a number of years older than Peter, and he had little emotional contact with them. But they retained more feelings for their father and saw more of him after his departure from the family home. Peter was left with his mother, who worked full-time. He described her as a sad, somewhat depressed woman, constantly tired, who had little to give him and resented any demands he made on her. Yet he felt sorry for her and tried, as any boy would in this situation, to make her feel good. It didn't work, but it left Peter with the feeling that something was demanded of him that he could not provide.

The closed-off quality in Peter's personality was apparent in his body, which was exceedingly tense. His jaw was tight, and his eyes were narrowed. Most significant, however, was his over-inflated chest, which looked as if it contained a great sorrow. Fortunately, when Peter did the breathing exercises, he broke down quickly into sobs. He felt the tragic quality of his life as well as his mother's. Crying released some of the sadness, and he felt better for it, but it didn't resolve his conflicts. Peter kept locked inside his tense upper back an enormous hostility toward women. He felt burdened by their sadness and helplessness and criticized for his inadequacy. I encouraged him to hit the bed in the therapy room and to express some of his anger toward his wife and his mother. "Leave me alone," he would say. "I'm not your slave, I can't provide for you, I'm angry at you, I could kill you." The more anger he expressed, the better he felt. It allowed him to feel that he might be free, that he could be a man, and that he wasn't obligated to be a "stud" for his wife. He would respond to her when he had the desire.

It is true that Peter's lack of interest in his wife may have been a way to withhold affection. Such behavior is similar to the action of a child who won't eat his food to spite his mother. Spiteful behavior is an indirect expression of anger and is used when direct expression is forbidden. Peter sometimes had an erection when he lay next to his wife, but when she responded with interest, he would lose it. That he recognized the spiteful nature of this action did not, however, eliminate it. To stop the spite, he had to express the underlying anger. I encouraged him to stand up to his wife, which he did from time to time. Strangely, whenever they had a fight, his sexual potency increased, and their relationship improved. However, he felt guilty about his self-assertion and his anger. This guilt had a sexual origin.

Peter related that his mother had a habit when she came home from work of sprawling on the living-room sofa with her legs apart, exposing her crotch. As he passed her, his eyes would invariably be drawn to this part of her body. But when she caught him looking at her, she gave him such a dirty look that he withdrew inwardly. This happened quite often, since he could not resist looking. He was ashamed of himself, especially since he developed sadistic and pornographic sexual fantasies as a result of his pent-up excitement. These fantasies made him feel dirty and confirmed his mother's disapproving look. But he could not get angry at her, because he was dependent on her, he felt sorry for her, and he felt that he was the transgressor. He was trapped, and he closed off to hide his shame. Unable to get back at his mother for exciting him, then putting him down, he got back at his wife by withholding sexual feeling.

This analysis helped free up Peter's anger, which he expressed more strongly in therapy and more openly at home. His wife's reaction was positive. She decided to go into therapy herself to work out some of her problems; earlier, she had placed the entire blame for her unhappiness on him. Their relationship continued to improve as Peter opened up. His situation at work also improved dramatically.

In my opinion, most men are afraid of women. Generally, they are not aware of this fear any more than they are aware of their hostility. They may say that they enjoy sex, but if they have unconscious negative feelings about women, they will not be able to give themselves fully in sex, and their pleasure will be limited.

Many men are engaged in power struggles with their partners. They see women as demanding and controlling and believe that to be committed to a love relationship entails a loss of personal freedom. Such men justify extramarital affairs as an assertion of their freedom. In some cases, these feelings may be justified, but even so they are the feelings of a child who experienced his mother as controlling. Having repressed the memory of those childhood experiences, men project onto their spouses the anger they felt at their mothers. All this takes place on an unconscious level, which is why the conflicts between husbands and wives are so difficult to resolve.

It helps to point out that a real man can't be dominated or controlled by a woman. Is he not her equal? If so, why can't he hold his own? A man's inability to stand up to a woman suggests that he sees her as a mother figure. If he complains that she castrates him, it is safe to assume that his mother castrated him already. A woman can castrate a child, but she cannot castrate a real man.

In cases like these, it pays to look at a man's childhood history to learn why and how he suffered a loss of manhood. Inevitably, his fear of women can be traced to the heartbreak he experienced as a child in relation to his mother. The process of analysis aims to help him free himself from the fixations that bind him to the past so that he can live more fully in the present.

Some men are overtly cruel and sadistic in their treatment of women. Instead of holding in their negative and angry feelings, they act them out. Generally, they fly into a rage at some minor frustration. It may seem that such an outburst is an expression of anger, but there is an important difference between anger and rage. The expression of anger is a constructive action aimed at restoring good feelings in a relationship. Rage, however, has a destructive effect; its aim is to control another person. It stems from frustration, not from hurt feelings, and it often involves a denial of power, which explains why it is so often vented on an inferior. [1]

A few men can stand up to women in a direct, self-assertive way. Such men are capable of feeling deep affection and security in their relationships, attitudes they express in the sexual act by neither ejaculating prematurely nor holding back.

The passive man, on the other hand, tends to be premature. The tension in his body, which results from the need to suppress his negative feelings, reduces his ability to stay with his excitement as it builds. He can no more yield to his sexual excitement than he can to the anger he holds for his mother and all other women. Is prematurity a way for such a man to get back at his partner by robbing her of satisfaction? Perhaps, but his own satisfaction is correspondingly reduced. A more correct interpretation of prematurity is as an expression of fear—the fear of standing up to a woman as the excitement mounts.

The hostile man, meanwhile, maintains erective potency by delaying his ejaculation, which gives him a sense of power. In this unconscious maneuver, the erect phallus is seen as a weapon with which to dominate and punish a woman. To delay the climax is also seen as a way not to give in. The effect of this maneuver is to reduce the man's pleasure and satisfaction. It also decreases his partner's pleasure, since her excitement is geared to and partly dependent on his.

Many men try to hold back their ejaculation deliberately to allow their partners to reach a climax. This is often accomplished by distracting the mind from sex, thereby decreasing the excitement. Such a maneuver rarely proves to be satisfactory to either party. Generally, a woman in this situation has to work to reach her climax because the overall level of excitement is low. The man, for his part, gets little out of this act of sex, though he may think, often mistakenly, that he has satisfied his partner. Unconsciously, the man sees the woman as a monster who, if she is not satisfied, could destroy him. Holding back his ejaculation is like holding in feelings. It adds enormous stress to the relationship and predisposes the man to heart disease. It also parallels the act of coitus interruptus, in which the man must curb his excitement so that he can control his response.

To love a woman is to enjoy her. Turn the statement around and it is equally true. To enjoy a woman is to love her. But no man can enjoy a woman if he is afraid of her, feels a need to control or dominate her, or has angry and hostile feelings toward her. If a man is afraid of a woman, he will serve his partner; if he is hostile and sadistic, he will demand that she serve him. But love is not an act of self-sacrifice. Nor is it something one gives. Instead, love comes from who one is: a loving person.

Women fear love much the same as men do. As children, they are subject to the same heartbreak as boys, and are caught equally in the power play between their parents, being pulled to one side or the other to serve their parents' needs. Most often, as we have seen, a girl is seduced by her father into an alliance against her mother. She is thus placed in a competitive position with her mother, who is stronger than she is. As a consequence, she looks to her father for protection. If he provides it, she will become trapped in a dependent relationship and end up as "daddy's little girl." If he doesn't protect her because he is afraid of his wife and feels guilty about his seductive behavior, she will feel betrayed. In that case, she will turn to her mother and become mama's little girl.

As adults, daddy's little girls are seductive with men and sensitive to their needs, just as they were with their fathers. Their role, as they see it, is to "be there" for men. Mama's little girls take the opposite role. Having been betrayed by their fathers, they feel angry and hostile to men. However, these roles can and do shift. The woman who plays the role of the sensitive and loving daughter to the man who appears strong and fatherlike may become denigrating and critical when he reveals the little-boy side of his nature. She may also be very supportive of a man in need but only by feeling superior. Poor boy, she might think, he needs mothering. By the same token, the tough, aggressive female may act like a little girl when she needs affection.

Sally was an attractive woman of about forty when she came to see me at the urging of friends. She had tried est and a number of other therapeutic modalities in search of something she could not name. She had her own successful business and several men who were interested in her. She might have married any number of men she didn't really want. The men she did want were not interested in marrying her.

Meeting Sally in her business or social life, one would not think she had a problem. She was vivacious, seemed happy, and mixed easily. But if one watched her carefully, it became apparent that her behavior was a facade. When she wasn't smiling or being gay, her face was drawn and her eyes were without feeling. She gave the impression of being a lost person whose facade was intended to hide her great sadness from others and from herself. Her body revealed a deep split in her personality. She had a very narrow waist, which separated her body into two dissimilar halves. The lower part of her body was full and well shaped but without much charge, so that it looked passive. Her breathing did not extend into her belly. The upper half of her body was narrow and small, with well-developed breasts. Her neck was rather thin and long so that her head did not seem well connected to her thorax. Clearly, her head was not connected to her heart, and her heart was not connected to her genitals.

Sally's relationship with men was somewhat unusual. She gave to them sexually, and showered them with gifts and help. As a result, men used her. Yet this did not make her angry with them, because it was what she expected. Was her behavior love or some form of self-sacrifice? To answer that, we need to examine her relationship with her father, to whom she had been very much attached. According to her own report, she would have done anything for him. She admired him greatly. He had been badly injured in the war but had made a remarkable recovery and become a successful attorney. Just as he was the light in her eyes, she was the apple of his. However, as an adult, her eyes lacked spark. What really had gone on between them?

Sally had an older brother who was attached to their mother but less deeply than Sally was to her father. She and her mother were not close. Sally saw her as immature and dependent and felt herself to be superior in almost every way. In the course of her analysis she stated many times that her mother had not been there for her. I could see that Sally's face was tight, her breathing shallow, and her voice constricted, all of which indicated a deprivation of nurturing by her mother during the first two years of life. Lying on the couch and reaching out with her arms brought up some very painful feelings. She remarked, "It's no use. I'll never get it," the "it" referring to love. Then she began to cry softly. At a deep level, Sally felt despair. As the therapy progressed, the feeling of despair became even stronger. On a number of occasions she exclaimed, "I don't want to live." Her facade had crumbled. Painful as this was, it was a necessary step in her struggle to regain her self.

Sally claimed that her father had loved her, which explained her attachment to him. But if his interest in her had been unselfish, she would have had a positive sense of herself as a person. Unfortunately, his love for her had been tainted with sexual interest. As we explored this aspect of her life, she admitted that she had been aware of that interest. Much as she had loved him, she had not wanted to be alone with him in the house. He had tried on a number of occasions to kiss her on the mouth, and once he had tried to get in bed with her, which had frightened her greatly. As she grew up and began to go out with boys, he became upset with her. Girls who were easy with boys, he had told her, were whores.

How could Sally handle her sexuality when it was stimulated by her father's interest and condemned by his puritanism? Instead, she dissociated herself from it. As a result, she could not identify with the lower part of her body. She was compulsively clean and said many times that the lower part of her body was dirty. And yet Sally came across as a very sexual woman; most men were strongly attracted to her. The shapeliness of the lower part of her body denoted her potential for sexuality, while the fact that it was held tightly, passively, and without feeling manifested her fear of surrender. Though Sally had many men, she had never had an orgasm. In discussing her sexual life, she said, "I'm a virgin whore."

Did Sally love men? Yes and no. Her relationship with men paralleled her relationship with her father. He was there for her in some nurturing capacity, and she was there for him in terms of the excitement between them. But she was not "there" for herself sexually. This was taboo, because it would turn her into a real tramp, not the whore who was still a virgin. She loved men because they were a source of excitement and life, but she also hated them because they used her, sullied her, and humiliated her, just as her father had. And because she allowed herself to be used and had even encouraged it as a child and later as a woman, she also hated herself.

Sally was not the rigid type. Her chest was relatively soft; her body, flexible. She was not just heartbroken; she was crushed to the point where she had almost no sense of self, no feeling that she had the right to demand or even ask for what she wanted. In psychiatric terms, she could be described as a borderline personality.[2] Her sense of self was very tenuous, and could easily be lost. One could also say that Sally's heart was open. As a result, she was not prone to coronary artery disease like the rigid, armored type. She did not struggle to win love, for she had no belief that she would ever be loved for herself. However, she did need some contact with men; otherwise, she would have felt utterly alone.

Since Sally's heart was open, it is fair to say that she had some love in her heart for the men with whom she was involved. But that feeling was limited to her heart and did not extend into her body. If she had loved these men with her body as well as her heart, she would have enjoyed the sexual contact with them and experienced some degree of orgasmic pleasure.

The problem for the rigid character is to open his heart fully to love. The problem for Sally was to become a person with a sense of self. That entailed a double approach: to open up her longing, which would allow her to discharge her sadness through crying, and to help her feel and express her anger at her father's betrayal. This anger also came out against the men who used her as an adult. That they used her with her permission didn't change the underlying anger. By expressing it, she began to reclaim her sexuality and to infuse the lower part of her body with life, a process she aided and abetted through deep breathing and appropriate exercises. Only when her sexuality was a fact in her being could she say that she truly loved men.

Women who love men feel no sense of inferiority or superiority to men and harbor no resentment or hostility toward them. All their experiences with the opposite sex as they grew up were positive. Not only their fathers but their brothers and other male relatives treated them with respect and affection, and their parents refrained from using them as pawns. Such an attitude toward a child, female or male, is only possible when there are no power struggles in the home, when love and respect are the dominant attitudes toward all members of the family, and when the overall mood is one of pleasure and good feeling. To put it simply, healthy children are the product of loving parents. But it is not enough for parents to love their children; more importantly, they must love each other. Such parents are fulfilled sexually with each other. Girls who grow up in homes where their parents fulfill each other sexually become women who respond orgasmically to the men they love.

One of the unfortunate consequences of the feminist movement has been its tendency to encourage women to blame men for their lack of fulfillment and sense of inferiority. Such a reproach to the male sex is not warranted. We have seen throughout this book that men are no more fulfilled in love and sexuality than women are. In terms of their vulnerability to heart disease and to early death, they are the weaker sex. It cannot be denied that they are stronger in such areas as politics, business, and the professions, all of which involve the acquisition and use of power. That power has often been used against women. But it is important to recognize that the possession of power and its use has not promoted the well-being of men. They have not loved more, lived longer, or had more joy because of it. In any relationship, the use of power harms the user as much as it does the person who is subject to it. As we have seen, power is destructive to love.

The issue between the sexes is one of equal respect, not one of equal power. What this means is that a woman should be treated with the same consideration as a man. Equal pay for equal work is her natural right as a person. Unfortunately, the phrase *equal work* is misleading. We are familiar with the idea that a woman executive should receive the same pay as a man in the same position. But what about the woman in charge of a nursery school? Is her work any less important? Shouldn't she be paid the same as any other person who shoulders important responsibilities? And the woman who stays home raising a family—is her work inferior? If we measure value solely in terms of money, we introduce power into all human relationships.

If women pursue power to the same degree that men have, they will fall heir to the same illnesses that have shortened men's lives. Fortunately, women are protected to some degree from this danger by their natural function as childbearers. So far in our history the drive in women to bear children has been stronger than the drive for power. But a woman's fulfillment lies not just in bearing children but in loving them. Here, too, nature has given her an advantage over the male sex, for she can express her love for her children more directly than a man through the act of nursing. Just as women who nurse babies are less prone to develop breast cancer, it is believed that they are less vulnerable to heart disease.

Broadly speaking, women are less afraid of love than men. They are less afraid to show emotions, less afraid of being tender, less concerned with their image. Women can cry more easily than men, partly because, as boys, men were pressured to be strong. A prohibition against breaking down may have made sense when men were hunters and warriors whose primary role was to protect the tribe. But rigidity in the face of a loss is not the same thing as bravery in a situation of danger. To hold back one's tears and sobs when a loved person dies is not an act of bravery but one of self-destruction.

By nature and conditioning men have always been the physically stronger sex. But strength does not have to mean toughness or rigidity. Tenderness is an asset to a man, just as it is to a woman, though for him it may be harder to come by. Still, the man who cannot melt the defenses he has erected to protect himself from hurt will never love. Moreover, as we shall explore in some detail in the following section, it is this lack of love that causes heart disease.

PART TWO

Heartbreak and Heart Disease

In the preceding chapters we studied the nature of love and examined its direct connection to the heart. We saw that many people in our culture suffer a loss of love in childhood that leaves them brokenhearted. In the interests of survival, they suppress the pain by armoring themselves—in other words, by rigidifying the muscles in the chest wall. This rigidification restricts and limits breathing, movement, and feeling, imposing a continuous stress on the body and the heart. It is the existence of this sort of stress, in my opinion, that predisposes so many people to heart disease.

In the second half of this book, we will explore the relationship between heartbreak and heart disease. We will pay special attention to the heart attack in an attempt to understand why it occurs when it does. To the psychologist or analyst viewing a person's life, a major illness is not a random event but one related to the individual's life-style. We will investigate some of the forces that shape that life-style and suggest ways in which they can be dealt with to create a life relatively free from severe stress. The bottom line, we will see, is this: Only the person who is not afraid to love can be reasonably secure that his heart will remain healthy.

CHAPTER 6

Love, Stress, and the Heart

Today most people accept the concept that undue stress can lead to illness. Such a general idea, however, does not offer much help in explaining a specific illness like coronary artery disease. Why would stress seriously damage the heart in one person while it produces arthritis in a second and cancer in a third? To put it differently, what is the nature of the stress that adversely affects the heart, and what kind of people are particularly vulnerable to heart disease if placed under such stress? Meyer Friedman and Samuel Rosenman addressed the second part of this problem when they began their pioneering research into the causes of coronary artery disease. That research, as they described it, was aimed at answering two questions: "First, can a person's feelings or thoughts have any influence upon the development of coronary artery disease? Second, if there is such a relationship, how does it work?"[1]

As a first step, these cardiologists studied their heart patients to see what characteristics distinguished them from other people. "As we looked at our patients in this new way, as individuals who possessed other organs than ailing hearts and also personalities," Friedman said, "it became obvious that it was not simply their hearts that had gone awry. Something in the way they felt, thought and acted was also in alarming disarray."[2] Almost all coronary patients, they observed, showed a similarity in their facial expressions, bodily gestures, and speech. A tight jaw and tight mouth muscles were characteristic, together with a tense body posture; rapid finger tapping or knee jiggling; fist clenching during ordinary conversation; teeth grinding; rapid body movements; rapid speech and impatience with the slow speech of others; and a snarllike grimace at the corners of the mouth, partially exposing the teeth.

These people also responded in a similar way to the events of daily life: They were very competitive, with an intense urge to win; they were easily irritated when others differed with them; they had fixed and angrily defended opinions; they were impatient when held up in traffic or waiting in line; they were compulsive to get things finished, so they ate quickly and walked quickly; and they could not tolerate inactivity.

Friedman and Rosenman labeled people who showed some or all of these traits Type A individuals and those free of these traits Type B individuals. They described the Type A individual as extremely tense, suffering from a sense of time urgency, harboring free-floating hostility of which he was unconscious, and struggling with low self-esteem, for which he compensated by achieving.

Friedman and Rosenman applied this classification to fifty-five hundred healthy men—that is, men with no history of heart disease, whom they followed for a period of eight and one-half years. At the end of the study, they noted that Type A men were seven times more likely to have coronary artery disease than their Type B counterparts. They also smoked more, had higher blood cholesterol levels, and were three times as likely to succumb to heart attacks. The study was so convincing that it dispelled any doubt of a direct relationship between attitudes, behavior, and heart disease. Further studies by others showed a similar result. Then Friedman went one step further. He reasoned that if Type A behavior could be modified, it should affect the individual's vulnerability to a subsequent heart attack. Such an outcome would constitute definitive proof that Type A behavior itself is a causative factor in coronary artery disease. This second study, extending over a period of three years, involved a number of patients with coronary artery disease who had suffered a myocardial infarction. The subjects were divided into three sections: The section I subjects were advised and followed by cardiologists; those in section II were given continued counseling about Type A behavior in small groups in addition to the treatment given those in Section I; and those in section III were simply followed.

When the data showing rates of recurrence were analyzed on a yearly basis, it was found that the "difference in recurrence rates between subjects in sections I and II the first year was 48 percent; in the second year, it was 62 percent, and in the third year it was *372 percent*."[3] By the end of three years, the difference was beyond any statistical challenge. Friedman explained these results by the fact that the subjects in section II showed a 30 percent reduction in Type A behavior.

And so the first of the two questions Friedman and Rosenman had asked was answered affirmatively: A person's feelings and thoughts do influence the development of heart disease.

This study involved a male-only population, since at the time it was done, the incidence of heart disease was greatly higher among men. Recent investigations, however, have shown increasing incidence of heart disease in women, especially in the last decade.[4] Type A behavior has become a fact of life for women, as well.

Friedman and Rosenman's second question, about the mechanics of the relationship between a person's subjective state and the development of heart disease, has been harder to answer.

Their studies have shown that Type A individuals have difficulty metabolizing the fat in their blood, whether they are healthy or already have heart disease. It has also been shown that Type A individuals have higher levels of norepinephrine, the "struggle hormone," in their blood. In addition, they secrete more ACTH, the hormone that stimulates the adrenal gland to produce the cortisonelike stress hormones, and less pituitary growth hormone than normal, while they overreact to sugar by producing excessive amounts of insulin. (This is consistent with the observation that the development of diabetes in maturity is a risk factor in coronary artery disease.) Experimental work with rats has also suggested that hostility may play a role. When the animals' emotional state is changed from peaceful to fiercely hostile by electrical stimulation of an area in the hypothalamus, they react just the way Type A individuals do: with increased levels of blood cholesterol, greater production of norepinephrine, and higher blood pressure.

A number of other studies have suggested that hostility may be the determining factor in the development of heart disease. Dombroski et al.,[5] reanalyzing data from structured interviews with coronary patients in one angiographic sample, found that "high levels of potential for hostility and 'anger-in' "—in other words, suppressed anger—"were strongly correlated with increased severity of coronary atherosclerosis (CAD)." In a study[6] of 255 physicians who had completed the Minnesota Multiphasic Personality Inventory while in medical school, those whose hostility scores were above the median showed a fivefold to sixfold higher rate of heart attacks and total mortality over a twenty-five-year follow-up period. But if we accept that hostility or held-in anger may be the prime element in causing coronary artery disease, we are still faced with the problem of explaining why it affects the heart, which is not an organ directly involved in the emotions of hostility and anger. Even if these emotions do produce an excess of norepinephrine, why does the heart become its specific target in some individuals?

To answer this question, we need to know that norepine-phrine acts to mobilize all the organs of the body, including the heart, to meet a threat or a crisis. If a person acts appropriately to meet the crisis, the hormone, having served its purpose, has no deleterious effects on any part of the body. But held-in anger keeps a person in a crisis situation *all* the time, which no amount of norepinephrine can discharge. The heart is put in the situation of being constantly stimulated but unable to act.

But most people in our culture have some degree of sup-pressed anger. At what point does it become life threatening? In order to answer this question, we need a different approach to the problem of heart disease, for the studies that have been done, valid as they are, leave too many gaps in our understanding of the disorder. After all, not every Type A individual develops coronary artery disease, nor do all Type B individuals escape it. In the Western Collaborative Group Study from which Fried-man and Rosenman drew their data, only 10 percent of the subjects diagnosed as Type A individuals suffered a heart attack in the eight and a half years of the study. Certainly more would have suffered an attack in time, but if time is a factor, we need to know how it operates.

Why does an attack occur when it does? In addition to such predisposing factors as Type A behavior, smoking, and high blood pressure, we must also take into account precipitating causes. In other words, what immediate stress in an individual's life is likely to trigger an attack? And what is the relationship of the precipitating cause to the predisposing factors? It has been reported that the loss of a job frequently acts as a precipi-tating cause of a heart attack. The loss of a loved person by death can also trigger a fatal heart attack, even in a person with no prior history of heart disease. Since the heart is implicated in love but not directly in hostility and anger, it is reasonable to think that disturbances in love are at the base of heart disease. In that case, an immediate crisis in an individual's love life may be a main factor in precipitating a heart attack. I believe we need to shift our focus in studying the whole problem of heart disease to the critical role that love—or the absence of love—plays in the health of the heart.

Friedman[7] himself has come to the conclusion that a lack of love is responsible for Type A behavior. "We now believe," he has written, "that one of the most important influences fostering insecurity is the failure of the Type A person in his infancy and early childhood to receive *unconditional love*, affection and encouragement from one or both parents." In this situation, the Type A individual has but one choice: to engage in "a continuous struggle, an unremitting attempt to accomplish or achieve, more and more—in less and less time."[8]

James Lynch has also suggested that a lack of love can cause heart disease.[9] In his book *The Broken Heart*, Lynch cites statistics that clearly show that married persons have a lower incidence of heart attacks than those who are single, divorced, or widowed. "At all ages, for both sexes, and for all races in the United States," he writes, "the unmarried always have higher death rates, sometimes as much as five times higher than those of married individuals." While this statement is true for all types of death, it has particular validity for deaths from cardiovascular disease. Lynch refers to studies that show a marked rise in death rates during the first six months following the loss of a loved one.[10] In 75 percent of the cases studied, death was caused by coronary artery disease, a fact that documents the damaging effect the loss of love can have on the heart. Not infrequently, the shock of the loss resulted in sudden death, often from a massive heart attack or ventricular fibrillation. We will examine the phenomenon of sudden death in a subsequent chapter.

What motivated Lynch to study the "medical consequences of loneliness" was his and others' observation that human contact can have a positive effect on the hearts of animals studied in labs as well as the hearts of patients in coronary care units. The entrance of a man into a laboratory room, for example, has been shown to excite a dog and increase its heart rate, while petting has been shown to calm the animal and reduce its heart rate significantly.[11] Human contact also affects the flow of blood in the coronary arteries. In some dogs, human contact has been demonstrated to be almost as potent an influence as strenuous exercise. Pulse taking, a seemingly routine human contact, has also been shown to have a strong effect on coronary care patients. Lynch reports: "In some of the patients, . . . pulse-taking had the power to completely suppress arrhythmias that had been occurring."[12] By the same token, studies have shown that petting a dog can reduce blood pressure in the person doing the petting.

The inescapable conclusion from these studies is that human beings need some loving contact. Many people look for such contact in marriage, but not all of them find it. Because of their fear of love, spouses often treat each other as adversaries and engage in power struggles. Thus we find that while married individuals are not as vulnerable to heart disease as those who live alone, they are not spared their heart attacks.

As Lynch observes, "There is . . . sufficient evidence available for us to anticipate a connection between marital discord and the development of coronary heart disease and premature death." He refers to a study by Dr. J. A. Medalne that followed ten thousand Israeli males with no evidence of heart disease for a period of five years. Those who later suffered a heart attack reported more problems in and dissatisfaction with their married life than the others. Yet all such a study tells us is that marital discord is a risk factor, not a determining one. Not all men in the study whose marriages were difficult suffered heart attacks. It's fair to assume, therefore, that some men coped better with the stress of marital discord than others.

A study done by Dr. Stewart Wolf,[13] a cardiologist, of the inhabitants of the town of Roseto, Pennsylvania, in the 1960s, demonstrated that the instability of emotional relationships creates stress that can have a damaging effect on the heart. Roseto is a town of about 1,630 people, mostly Italian, located about sixty miles from New York City. Wolf was drawn to it in the first place because its inhabitants suffered only one-third as many heart attacks as people in surrounding communities although their diet and their cholesterol levels were about the same. What protected these people against heart disease? The most significant difference, Wolf noted, was the quality of Roseto's community life. The family was the focus of daily life, and the town's inhabitants still lived according to the social customs and traditions that had prevailed in their former homeland. This focus on maintaining the integrity of family relationships favored a style of life that avoided conflict and marital discord.

Unfortunately, the town underwent a dramatic change in the two decades following the study. Industry moved in, new homes were built, and Roseto enjoyed a prosperity unknown before. The effect in most people's lives was to change the home from being the center of life to a base they left in the morning and returned to at night. It wasn't long before the vital statistics of health and disease showed that Roseto had become like its neighbors, with an incidence of heart disease and heart attacks no different from theirs.

The family stability that once characterized Roseto is quite rare today and cannot be created by will or decree. Many of us live with the stresses of marital conflict and the actual or threatened breakup of relationships as a fact of modern life. It is important to understand the nature of these stresses if we are to cope with them effectively.

It seems from the studies described above that two different types of stress can affect the heart. One stems from stressful situations in the world, most often in the workplace, and is associated with Type A behavior. The other stems from situations in the home, where it is associated with marital discord and a lack or loss of love. But are these situations unrelated? We have noted that Type A behavior is motivated by a need for greater self-esteem, a need that can be traced back to a lack of

unconditional love in childhood. However, we need unconditional love even as adults. It seems unlikely that those who
experience its richness would succumb as easily to stress as those
who don't. Given the central role of love in our lives, it is
unfortunate that Friedman and Rosenman did not investigate
the love lives of their subjects as thoroughly as they observed
their overt behavior.

Though situations of marital discord lead so often to hostility, they don't need to. The alternative is for spouses to have a
good fight. Certain conflicts can be discussed and resolved
calmly, but not those that have to do with the deeper issues of
power and self-esteem that trouble most marriages. A woman
may feel, for example, that her husband uses her, ignores her
feelings, or humiliates her. A man may feel burdened by his
wife's dependency, put down by her critical comments, or put
off by her lack of sexual desire. Resentments like these lead to
hostility if they are not expressed. But the expression of negative feelings generally evokes anger, which is all well and good
if the spouses are prepared to fight. Not all are. Many couples
are afraid to express their anger because it disturbs the relationship. One husband said, "I can't let any anger out because my
wife feels too threatened." Several women have reported that
when they become angry, their husbands withdraw. Other
people have difficulty even feeling angry because the emotion
was so deeply suppressed in childhood that it is unavailable to
them as adults. If, on the other hand, their parents constantly
fought, as mine did, they tend to avoid disputes and confronta-
tions because of the unpleasantness they create without necessarily resolving anything. My parents never vented their anger at
each other, which is why they were perpetually hostile. As a
result, I have had to work hard in my own therapy to make my
anger more available.

Is expressing anger stressful in itself? Many people believe
that all emotions are stressful and that the best way to avoid
stress is to stay calm, play it cool, and to let disturbing

situations slide off like water off a duck's back. But not to react requires an effort, since the natural tendency is to react. Human beings are sentient organisms whose responses to their environment are motivated by their feelings and guided by their thoughts. In most cases, behavior can be controlled by thinking and reason operating through the ego, but when feelings become very intense, they can override the ego's control, leading to actions that might otherwise be restrained. For example, an employee might become so angry at an insult by his boss that he will express his anger despite the threat it poses to his position. In such a case, to hold back the expression would take a considerable effort of will, which would constitute a stress to the body.

We can reduce feeling only by deadening ourselves or by developing a thick skin, which reduces not only the impact of the environment but also our ability to respond or reach out. Of course, this results in an insensitivity to positive forces as well as to negative ones, to love as well as to hostility. It might seem that such a protective maneuver would insulate us from the common stresses of life; in fact, the reverse is true. Such armoring taxes us and, by wearing us out, makes us even less resistant to stress.

To appreciate this paradox, consider the following: A man carrying a hundred pounds of flour or coal on his shoulders has to tense the appropriate muscles to support the load. That tension is visible in his raised shoulders and tight musculature and can be measured by an electromyograph, which records the amount of tension in the muscle. In order to maintain his balance, the tension must be equal to the hundred pounds of pressure exerted by the load. But the stress is not in the weight itself but in the tension in the muscles of the body.

Many people complain of emotional burdens, and their bodies show tensions similar to those imposed by physical weights. Their shoulders are raised, their backs are bowed, and their muscles are severely contracted, sometimes to the point of pain.

Emotional burdens are as powerful stressor agents as physical burdens and operate in much the same way. Unfortunately, it is often easier to get rid of a physical burden than an emotional one. The stress produced by the latter is generally longer lasting and more harmful to the body.

The body can cope very well with some measure of stress. We can carry some weight, support some degree of emotional burden, and consciously restrain our actions and impulses without any difficulty. However, when the burden is unremitting or the restraint chronic, the stress becomes damaging. The greater damage occurs when we are no longer conscious of the burdens we carry or the restraints we have imposed on ourselves because we no longer feel the tension in our body.

I am not arguing that the conscious restraint of behavior is unnatural or harmful. Quite the contrary. We often consciously control or modify our behavior so that it is appropriate to the situation at hand. The ability to respond effectively in this fashion is a function of self-possession. But before we can consciously control our actions, we must be aware of the feelings that motivate a particular response, and we must have the ability to express them. Self-possession, then, depends on self-awareness and self-expression. People who are relatively healthy are usually very self-possessed. In those who are neurotic, the unconscious control of behavior operates to reduce their self-possession. Such unconscious control is apparent in the difficulty they have in saying no, in asking for help, or in crying when hurt, or getting angry when insulted. It is also apparent in the amount of chronic muscular tension or rigidity in the body.

Rigidity is the main mechanism for the unconscious control of feeling. It is accomplished by tensing the voluntary muscles of the body so that impulses are denied their avenues of expression. To block an impulse to cry, the face is tightened; to restrain an impulse to strike out, the shoulders and back are tensed. When these tensions become chronic, the blocked impulse does not reach the surface of the body or consciousness.

Self-awareness has become limited. Rigidification amounts to a deadening of the body. Eventually, we become "stiffs." As I point out to patients, dead men have no feelings. When there is no spontaneous movement in the body, there is nothing to feel. Emotions are involuntary activities of the body. They happen *to* us. We do not desire to love someone, we fall in love. We are moved to tears or to anger. Emotions and feelings are not functions of the ego, which controls the voluntary actions, those subject to our will. Emotions are impulses arising at the core of our being, closely connected to the heart. We shall see that rigidity can, however, extend into the depths of an organism, affecting the smooth, involuntary muscles. One finds such spasticities in the smooth muscles of the intestines, the bronchi, and the arteries. When rigidity develops in the peripheral blood vessels, it causes hypertension, which places an enormous strain on the heart muscle and is a recognized risk factor for coronary artery disease. When it develops in the coronary vessels themselves, where it is associated with the formation of atheromatous plaques that narrow these vital supply lines, there is a serious risk of a fatal heart attack.

If we are to understand the role emotions play in producing stress, we must examine another mechanism for the unconscious control of feeling. That mechanism is known as denial. Denial doesn't operate by deadening the body but by blocking the perception of an impulse. A typical case of denial is the person who in a discussion starts to shout and yell but when asked if he is angry, angrily denies that he is.[14] Denial operates by dissociating the perceptual functions of the head and ego from the core functions of impulse formation. Actually, both mechanisms, denial and rigidity, exist in most individuals to varying degrees.

Denial accounts for the fact that many people who suppress their feelings also have a strong tendency to overreact. We noted earlier that when anger is suppressed, resentments build up. When they, too, are denied, the underlying anger smolders like a slumbering volcano, manifesting its existence by little puffs of steam—in the form of irritability or critical remarks—that escape through cracks in the crust. But in many of these people, continued frustrations can raise the energy of the inner fire to an explosive level, resulting in the breakthrough of an irrational and exaggerated response. Expressing their rage doesn't free them, because their reaction is so arbitrary it makes them feel guilty, which fans the flames of their hostility all over again.

One may wonder what connection rage has to heart disease, or for that matter, why holding anger in is so harmful to the heart. The answer is that anger is a constructive reaction, which includes some feeling of affection and love, whereas rage contains an element of hate. When we express our anger, we imply that we care for a person and that we want to restore the relationship to where love and friendship can be felt and expressed. We tend not to get angry at people who mean little to us because if their behavior is hurtful, we can walk away.

One of my patients reported on this positive aspect of anger. He had married his wife out of a feeling of loneliness. For her, he was a rebound from an earlier disappointment in love. For obvious reasons, their relationship never blossomed, and my patient suffered from depression. He escaped from this unhappy situation by throwing himself into his work. The amount of anger he held in was enormous, but he never expressed it. He felt guilty, and his self-esteem was so low that he believed he had no right to make a demand for love. It took more than a year of therapeutic work before his anger surfaced. The muscular tension in his body was also enormous, equal to the amount of suppressed anger. Much of this tension had to be released before he could get in touch with his feelings. At the same time, a careful analysis had to be done so that he could free himself from his guilt by understanding how his mother had created his problem by her treatment of him as a child. She had divorced his father because he had failed to measure up to her expectations. My patient became her "houseboy."

When his anger first surfaced, he felt he wanted to smash my office. I let him hit my bed (which was a five-inch foam mattress) from a standing position, which allowed him to discharge some of his rage without hurting himself or anyone else. He pounded the bed for several months. One day he came in and told me that he had gotten angry at his wife. She had come home at night and immediately began to watch a television show. He told her angrily that if she preferred watching TV to being with him, he would leave. I don't know how the argument progressed, but I do know that they made love that night, which was not common for them, and that, according to my patient, it was good.

I have heard similar stories from many patients over the years to the effect that a clean fight, with the open expression of anger between love partners, often ends in an act of love. On the other hand, when there is unexpressed anger between lovers, it is almost impossible to consummate a sexual union. Anger opens the heart because it says, in effect, "I care." Hostility, on the other hand, closes the heart, turning it cold to the other.

The hyperactive individual is identical in many respects to the Type A personality. He reacts to every situation of conflict and criticism as if it were a threat to his security and self-esteem. He is always on the defensive, which he covers up by a pseudoaggressiveness. Friedman's treatment of this behavior problem is to make the person aware of his state of tension, of his hyperactivity, and of his compulsive drive to achieve. Friedman points out correctly that this compulsive drive undermines creativity and so handicaps any productive efforts that it fails in the end to enhance the individual's self-esteem. To the degree that the hyperactive person responds to this treatment, he will feel more relaxed and less driven, which will relieve some of the stress on the heart. But there are problems with this approach. Not only does it fail to recognize the chronic muscular tensions from which the hyperactive individual suffers, it fails to get to the heart of the problem.

The heart of the problem is love, and the locus of the

problem is the home. The stresses of the workplace may be great, but they are manageable when a person is in a secure, stable, and loving relationship. It is what happens in the home that creates the stresses that most seriously affect the heart.

I know this from my own experience. My wife has often accused me of being hostile to her, and I have as often denied it. I've argued that I love her, and indeed I do, but I have resented her reluctance to declare her unconditional love for me. On occasions when I hurt her by some remark that I would say I did not mean, she pulled away from me and at times threatened to end our marriage. This threat frightened me and made me aware that I had some deep fear of abandonment. I felt hurt by her rejection, which made me more hostile to her. But I couldn't get angry at her wanting to leave me if she felt that my behavior wounded her and made her unhappy. But just as I hurt her by some critical or negative remark, she also hurt me by her criticism. I felt put down when she disparaged me by pointing out an instance of weakness or carelessness. I felt that she was treating me like my mother, who had admired me on the one hand but on the other made me aware that I wasn't measuring up to her expectations. When I pointed this out to my wife, she replied that I treated her as if she were my mother.

My problem as I see it now was that I didn't sense my hostility. When accused of it, I became defensive, which only increased it. But how could I be hostile to the person I loved and whose love I wanted, since by recognizing my hostility I would, I feared, destroy the possibility of getting that love? I felt trapped in this situation. Fortunately, I didn't panic, or stiffen up in self-defense. Instead, I tried to sense my feelings. I cried as I recognized a deep sadness. I had never felt the unconditional love I wanted so desperately, and I could sense how angry I was. I also realized that I did not want to live in a state of ambivalence. If I couldn't have the love I wanted, I would take my pain and leave. I would not stay trapped. I had to be free.

To be free meant I had to be true to myself. I could not continue to play the game of "you hurt me and I hurt you back." I decided I would not let my wife disparage me for any reason. I had my weaknesses just as she had hers. When she criticized me, she became my mother and I felt angry whether her criticism was justified or not. Most often it was justified, but that didn't excuse her saying it in a way that made me feel small. One evening during one of our set-tos, my anger flared, and I told her that I would hit her if she put me down again. My anger was so strong that I did not care what happened to our relationship. It's hard to be afraid when one is so angry. But it didn't break up our relationship. I was surprised to find that my wife reacted positively to this expression of anger. And I had a strong feeling of being set free. To be free of those negative feelings gave me such a feeling of lightness that I realized what a burden and stress they had been to me.

I believe we all want to be free, to love unconditionally, to give ourselves wholeheartedly in love and sex. Given the experiences of our childhood, it is not easy to reach this state. My anger at my mother for some of the cruel things she did to me had been suppressed. I recall an incident from the age of three. She was handling me roughly as she dressed me, and I began to strike her with my fists. She turned to me and with a look of reproach said, "How can you strike your mother?" She made me feel so terrible that I never hit her again, or anyone else except in self-defense. The implied threat in her words was that to strike someone you love is a major crime. I know I submitted, and my rebellion became insidious. But what else can a small child do? Over time, as I suppressed my anger, I experienced a buildup of severe tension in my upper back and around the shoulders. Eventually I became a typical candidate for a heart attack—a rigid, armored individual, with my head somewhat bowed, my back rounded, and my breathing restricted. But I have changed that through the work I have done with myself—a brief description of which follows.

Let me say that I have had enough therapy to become aware of the tensions in my body and the fears associated with them. My biggest fear was that of being abandoned if I didn't fulfill my parents' expectations. There was an element of panic in this fear, which I tried not to feel by keeping my body tense and rigid. I was also aware of a deep sadness relating to the loss of my mother's breast at an early age. This sadness shows in my earliest pictures. Even though I was aware of this sadness, crying was difficult. To me, crying meant breaking down and feeling helpless—a feeling I strongly resisted. The resistance was in the form of a stiff back and a stiff neck. I did intensive work with my body to soften it so crying would come through more easily. I did special grounding exercises to strengthen my legs so I could feel secure in them. I released much of the tension in my upper back by hitting the bed with my fists regularly while verbally expressing anger. (I will describe these exercises in chap. 10.) I want to emphasize that in most cases it is necessary to work with the body as well as with the mind to make the changes that would ensure a healthy heart.

CHAPTER 7

The Heart Attack

In this chapter we will look at the events immediately preceding a heart attack to determine the emotional state of the victim. We know that the stress associated with Type A behavior renders a person vulnerable to heart disease and a heart attack. That stress stems from the suppression of such feelings as hostility, longing, sadness, and fear—all of which are associated with the experience of heartbreak in early childhood. It is manifested in chronic muscular tensions, which result in an inflated chest, a tendency to hold the breath, shallow breathing, and overall rigidity. Stress also causes an increase in the production of adrenal hormones, disturbances in the metabolism of fatty acids, and reduced production of prostacycline. Let us examine these biochemical changes in some detail.

Normally, when a person faces a situation of stress or danger, the body mobilizes its energy to meet the stress or remove the danger. Many systems act together to promote this mobilization. The brain has two major nerve networks that regulate and control the body's reactions: the voluntary nervous system and the autonomic system. The first is concerned predominantly with the actions of the striated or voluntary muscles, which are largely subject to conscious control. The second, the autonomic system, is concerned with the operation of the organs, glands, and smooth muscles, all of which are normally beyond conscious control. The autonomic system has two opposing parts, the parasympathetic and the sympathetic. The parasympathetic coordinates the organism's response to pleasurable stimuli. It acts to relax and expand the body. When the stimuli are threatening or painful, the sympathetic system acts to contract the body and mobilize its defenses. An example of this antagonistic action is seen in the effect of these two systems on the heart; the parasympathetic slows down the heart rate, and the sympathetic speeds it up. The latter action helps the heart deliver more blood to the muscles when they are actively engaged in coping with a threatening situation.

In addition to this nervous regulation, various glands secrete hormones that play an active role in the mobilization of the body's defenses. Prominent among them are the adrenal glands, which secrete hormones known as catecholamines. Two of these hormones, adrenaline and norepinephrine, increase heart activity, raise the blood pressure, and constrict peripheral blood vessels, bringing more oxygen and nutrients to the brain, the heart, and other muscles. We all know what a boost adrenaline provides to someone under great stress. The catecholamines also influence the metabolism of fat, the body's storehouse of energy, by producing free fatty acids that become transformed in the liver into triglycerides. But the action of these hormones has also been implicated in heart disease. The lipoproteins that result may be deposited on the walls of arteries to form atheromatous plaques, which narrow the arteries and reduce or block the flow of blood. When this narrowing occurs in the coronary arteries, it becomes one of the factors responsible for a heart attack. The other factor is coronary spasm, which, acting upon a sclerotic artery, will completely cut off the flow of blood to the heart muscle.

This simple analysis raises an important question. Why should a mechanism that nature designed to help an organism react to a threat to its integrity turn out to be one of the causes of disease? The answer is that damage results when the body is mobilized to act but fails to because it is frozen by fear. When an organism responds to a threat by fighting or fleeing, heightened physical activity uses up the extra energy that the metabolism of fat makes available. But in a situation of stress or danger, in which neither of these actions is possible, the excess lipoproteins will be deposited on the arterial walls.

Two situations illustrate clearly what happens on a metabolic level when a person is trapped and cannot respond effectively to stress. It has been found that the blood cholesterol level of accountants rises sharply as the stress of preparing tax returns increases toward the April 15 deadline. They can neither fight nor flee, but have to sit at their desks until their work is done. The same elevated cholesterol levels have been found in medical students during examination periods. They, too, are temporarily trapped by a situation that requires submission to stress. For both accountants and medical students, the degree of stress experienced depends on the state of the individual. Those who are more relaxed will feel less stress, while those who are frightened will suffer more severe stress.

One other system is relevant to our study. This one involves the production of compounds that control the viscosity of the blood. These compounds are thromboxane (TxA_2) and prostacycline ($P61_2$), both derived from arachic acid, which is present in vessel walls and in blood plasma. The action of these compounds is antagonistic; thromboxane causes the aggregation of blood platelets and is the most potent agent in causing blood vessels to contract. Prostacycline inhibits platelet aggregation and dilates the blood vessels. Under normal conditions the blood flows freely through the arteries. To facilitate this flow, prostacycline coats the lining of the arteries so that nothing sticks. But when the wall of an artery is damaged, thromboxane, produced from the damaged tissue, causes the platelets to stick together like a clot at the same time that the artery contracts. This action prevents or diminishes hemorrhaging and is one of the body's important defense mechanisms. The catecholamines, or "struggle hormones," favor the production of thromboxane. But if the body produces an excess of thromboxane, clots may form on non-damaged arterial walls. An excess of thromboxane means a deficiency of prostacycline.

The Polish researcher R. Gryglewski[1] has furthered our understanding of these complex mechanisms by demonstrating that prostacycline is produced in the lungs. When subjects in his study were stimulated pharmacologically to breathe more, the level of prostacycline in their blood vessels rose. Other researchers have confirmed this finding. In view of this connection between breathing and the production of prostacycline, J. Santorski[2] describes the following sequence of events: STRESS $\longrightarrow$ BREATHING LIMITATIONS $\longrightarrow$ LESS PROSTACYCLINE $\longrightarrow$ SCLEROSIS. (It's no accident that oxygen is the first thing administered to a heart attack victim. If he had taken in enough oxygen during his life, he might have been spared the attack.)

The continued action of all these factors over years damages the coronary arteries, producing some degree of atherosclerosis. In this condition the coronary arteries stiffen, and their lumen (or functional width) is narrowed, reducing the flow of blood to the heart muscle. If this condition is severe in any one of the arteries, the individual so afflicted will experience pain in the region of his heart upon exertion—for example, climbing stairs. This pain, called angina, is a clear symptom of coronary artery disease, but an individual may suffer from angina for a long time without having a heart attack. On the other hand, he may have a severe heart attack without any previous experience of anginal pain.

A heart attack occurs when one of the coronary arteries closes down completely, depriving a section of heart muscle of necessary oxygen. The deprived muscle fibers die in a process known as myocardial infarction, often designated by the letters MI in the professional literature. If the infarction is extensive, the heart may go into shock or develop ventricular fibrillation, and the person may die. If the person survives the attack, some healing of the heart takes place. The dead muscle cells are replaced by fibrous tissue, forming a scar. A scarred heart is a damaged heart, but the extent of the damage depends on the location and extent of the infarction. After recovery from a heart attack, most people can lead relatively normal lives, and many will not suffer another heart attack. However, if the pressures and stress that culminated in the first attack are not reduced, there is a strong likelihood that a second or third attack will occur, with a fatal outcome.

Although it is necessary for only one of the coronary arteries to close down for an MI to occur, generally the others are not free from the disease. Cardiologists use angiograms—X-ray pictures of blood vessels made after the injection into the vessels of an opaque dye—to determine the extent to which the coronary arteries have narrowed. If the disease has progressed to the point where the arteries are handicapped in their function, a bypass operation may be recommended so that the diseased arteries may be replaced by clean veins. In this way a more normal blood flow is restored to the heart muscle. But if the conditions that led to the problem persist, these substitute "arteries" become damaged in time.

It is generally assumed that a heart attack occurs when the heart is subjected to an overwhelming stress. We are familiar with the fact that older men sometimes suffer heart attacks while shoveling snow. Tennis players, marathon runners, and other sports enthusiasts sometimes suffer them, as well. A classic example is the case of James Fixx, the author of several popular books on running, who died during a run. Later it was learned that he suffered from coronary artery disease. Obviously, he pushed himself too hard, and his heart couldn't take it. But neither shoveling snow nor running is inherently dangerous. Older men, like myself, often shovel snow without any ill effects, just as many men run or play tennis regularly without harm. It is the pushing and straining that are dangerous, because they are so often accompanied by some holding of the breath.

Actions resulting from spontaneous impulses are generally effortless. When a movement arises out of the feeling that inspires it, it has a unified quality: All parts of the body are freely coordinated in the action, and there is never a lack of oxygen. No effort is required, for example, for us to run to greet someone we haven't seen for a long time. Most commonly, however, our actions and movements are goal oriented and often require some exercise of the will to achieve the goal. Pushing or using the will tenses the muscles, which hinders respiration. When we are strongly focused on a goal, we may feel ourselves to be under such pressure to achieve it that we don't stop to breathe. On the other hand, by focusing on our breathing, we can greatly diminish the stress of any activity. In shoveling snow, for example, it is essential to stop to breathe regularly. Trying to overcome feelings of distress or tiredness is asking for trouble.

James Fixx could have saved his life if he had quit running when he sensed some distress. Quitting, however, would have been an admission of failure, which obviously was unacceptable. When failure is equated with a loss of self-esteem and, therefore, of the right to be loved, it can be overwhelming enough to result in feelings of helplessness and hopelessness, which can end in collapse.

For many men in our culture, the need to prove their manhood is a powerful drive. To be weak or helpless entails a tremendous loss of self-esteem. But to maintain an image of power, strength, and competence requires a tremendous investment of energy in a particularly harmful posture. To thrust out the chest, suck in the belly, straighten the shoulders, tighten the jaw, and stiffen the back might endow a man with a macho appearance, but it severely limits his breathing, at the same time rendering him insensitive to the physical and emotional stresses he subjects himself to.

But these are special cases. Most heart attacks do not occur during strenuous physical activity. One study of 1,347 attacks determined that only 2 percent occurred during physical exertion.[3] The question of the relationship of exertion to heart disease enters the picture most often when a physician counsels a postinfarction patient about his ability to perform coitus. Postinfarction patients commonly fear that such exertion could overstress the heart and result in another attack. But such anxiety is not limited to postinfarction males. Although a number of jokes about "death in the saddle" suggest that a heart attack during sex is the ideal way to exit this world, death rarely occurs during intercourse. In a Japanese study of thirty thousand deaths, only thirty-five were known to have occurred during sexual activity. Of these thirty-five, twenty-eight occurred while the man was having intercourse with a woman other than his wife. The implication is that it is not sexual activity that is the killer but guilt. One medical examiner noted that death in such circumstances usually occurs in unfamiliar surroundings after a big meal with alcohol. If the man involved is an older man, he may barely be able to perform at all. For him to push himself to avoid failing places him under enormous emotional and physical stress.

One can "overdo" it on many levels simultaneously. When this happens, the stresses are often more than the heart can support. The following case report illustrates this combination of stresses. A doctor whom we will call Arthur described the events surrounding his heart attack as follows:

> My father died at the age of thirty-eight from an acute infarction. I had an MI at the age of thirty-seven on Christmas

Day. The irony of this "gift" has not escaped me, nor the fact that I was following in my father's footsteps, albeit a year earlier.

At the time of my infarction I had recently split up with a lady that I had been seeing intermittently and gone back to another woman that I had had an unstable and explosive relationship with for some time. Perhaps one could best describe my love and sexual relationships as being immature and unstable. I was unable to "settle down," "make a commitment," and my sexual activity, with multiple partners, was rather compulsive. Yet I always returned to a generally unsatisfactory and emotionally explosive relationship with this particular woman. At the time of my infarction I had never had any cardiovascular symptoms (i.e., no angina, dysrhythmia, etc.) I would occasionally have my blood pressure taken at work in the emergency department, and for a few months prior to the infarction I had intermittently high diastolic pressures (110 range).

As a medically trained internist, I can say that the only risk factors (at least those recognized by our "mechanistic" orthodoxy) were family history, cigarette smoking, and a somewhat sedentary lifestyle. At the time of the event my serum cholesterol was in the 250 range.

The MI itself occurred after I had worked a string of nights in the emergency department (7:00 P.M. to 7:00 A.M.). I went home Christmas morning and awoke at one in the afternoon with a peculiar chest pain. It felt as if my chest were suspended by high tension wires pulling and tugging in different directions. It was uncomfortable, but it didn't exactly hurt. I remember wondering if I could be having an MI. I did note that the pain radiated down both arms and that I was perspiring heavily and slightly nauseated. Tensing my pectoral muscles made it somewhat worse. Thinking it was from muscular tension, I tried masturbating, but it only made the pain worse, and I wasn't able to have an orgasm. I got up, took a bath, and felt somewhat better, but "washed out." I thought I had a virus and proceeded to go out as planned for dinner with the woman I had been seeing and her family. I came home early. I went to work the day following Christmas at seven in the morning, even though I looked and felt terrible. Just before going home I decided on a "whim" to get a cardiogram on myself. I took one look at it and said, "Oh, fuck." I had had an acute inferior infarction. My subsequent hospitalization was stormy. I had five bypassed vessels; post-op my oxygen pressure plummeted, and I became—understandably—confused.

One more case of a man overdoing it, going all the way to prove his manhood and denying his body. The following report of the heart attack and death of a thirty-six-year-old man presents a similar scenario. The attack occurred while Joseph was on vacation in Florida with his wife. The vacation was his first break from work in over eight months from a very demanding and responsible job. He was very competent in his field, but the fact that he smoked three packs of cigarettes a day indicated the stress he was under. In addition, he was overweight and did little physical exercise. The day of the attack Joseph played eighteen holes of golf. That evening he and his wife went to a dinner show, where he had a fairly large meal. According to his wife, he forewent dessert, which he normally ate, and complained of some discomfort after the meal.

The couple returned home about midnight and engaged in sex. Joseph's wife related that his ejaculation was flat and that his body went limp at the climax. Immediately after, he again complained of some distress. He demurred when his wife suggested that she call a doctor, saying his discomfort would pass. But soon after he said his head felt funny, and he became pale. His wife said he looked as if he were stoned. She became seriously alarmed when he said he thought he was having an anxiety attack and called for an ambulance, but he was dead before the ambulance arrived.

Clearly, Joseph was a candidate for a heart attack. If he was as brilliant as his wife claimed, he should have known it. His behavior seemed to indicate that he went out of his way to challenge his vulnerability or, as we shall see in a subsequent chapter, to confront his fate. For many men, cigarette smoking is identified with manliness. To give up smoking, therefore, can be seen, on an unconscious level, as an admission of failure. Joseph was committed to success at all costs. He had to prove that he was a winner in his golf game, at dinner, and in sex. He pushed himself to the limit—and beyond—to fulfill his image. In the sexual act, he may have come face-to-face with his impotence and panicked.

Most men fear failure in sex, associated as it is with the loss of love. Until recently, that fear did not trouble women as much, but the situation is changing as more and more enter a competitive work world in which they are judged by their performance. Many develop Type A behavior, which predisposes them to heart disease. In the last two decades the incidence of coronary artery disease and myocardial infarction has risen dramatically among the female population. The change in their life-style also affects their sexual functioning. In a recent study of sexual dysfunction among women, 218 working and non-working wives were questioned at the Masters and Johnson Institute about their sexual responsiveness. The analysis of the data showed that women who were pursuing careers requiring a major commitment of time and energy were twice as likely to seek help for inhibited sexual desire as women employed in less demanding jobs or women unemployed outside the home.[4] Career women also had more complaints of vaginismus than the other two classes of women. For both men and women, then, this drive to perform places them under great pressure and at the same time it interferes with their ability to discharge that pressure through the pleasure and fulfillment of love.

A sixty-year-old woman executive whom we shall call Lucy had exactly these problems, but fortunately she retired before her condition deteriorated to the point where she developed heart disease. Lucy came to me depressed after she had been demoted at a large corporation. She blamed her demotion on the jealousy of her superior, but the official reason she was given was that she lacked judgment. Whatever the reason, it was not difficult to see that she was tense and driven. She was overweight and ashamed of her figure, and she commented that her cholesterol level was extremely high—over 300. I noticed that her jaw was tight, denoting that she had used considerable effort to reach her position, and that her chest was inflated and her breathing poor. The same strong will that had allowed her to rise in the business world was unavailable to her in her private life: She smoked about two packs of cigarettes a day, although she had tried many different ways to stop smoking. Simply stated, her problem was a need to prove her competence and superiority, a typical narcissistic disorder.

I believe Lucy was spared a heart attack because she accepted an early retirement after her demotion. In this way, she was relieved of the stress of a competitive situation. Her subsequent depression brought her into therapy, where she realized that corporate life was not her cup of tea and that her real desire was for a loving relationship with a man. She also stopped smoking. Thus, Lucy came to construe her failure as freedom. Had she not, she would have struggled to maintain her self-esteem, which would have placed her under continuing stress and pressure.

In *The Healing Heart*, Norman Cousins credits Arnold Hutshneves, author of *The Will to Live*, with the idea that "people who feel locked into obligations that they would rather set aside are candidates for sudden and severe disease."[5] Cousins himself suffered a heart attack at home after a return from "a hectic trip to the East Coast just before Christmas."[6] He was faced with the prospect of another trip to the Southeast in a few days, which he thought might be more than he could handle. However, he felt unable to cancel the engagement. The next day, he had a heart attack.

"Just after lunch," Cousins recounts, "I was hit by a wave of nausea and weakness. I began to pant. I had none of the massive, squeezing pains generally associated with a heart attack, but pressure in my chest and difficulty in breathing left little doubt that my heart was failing." Cousins's wife hooked him up to a portable oxygen tank until the paramedics arrived. From this point on, he made every effort to avoid panic, which he believes is the real killer. *The Healing Heart*, which describes his recovery from what was diagnosed as "significant" heart-muscle destruction and congestive heart failure, is an interesting account of the power of psychological and emotional factors to influence disease.

But can they cause disease? Cousins was not a typical Type A individual—he believed in laughter as the way to handle stress, he didn't smoke or drink, his blood pressure was low, and he wasn't overweight. He usually engaged heavily in sports but had eased off lately due to the pressure of travel. Two months earlier he had experienced shortness of breath in cold weather, a sensation of pressure in his throat, heaviness in his right leg, and there were some traces of blood in his sputum. However, an EKG showed no pathology, and the symptoms receded. Nevertheless, something was wrong. Unfortunately, most physicians cannot see a disease process until it leads to structural pathology. No one checked to see how well or how poorly Cousins breathed, how rigid his body was, how inflated his chest, how tight his throat, how tense his jaw. If we wish to understand illness, especially chronic illness, we must use a holistic approach and look at the person as well as his organs.

The idea that unwanted obligations can lead to serious illness is suggestive but incomplete. If the situation evokes feelings of panic and helplessness, it could certainly be dangerous, especially if the feelings go unrecognized. The effort to block the expression of such feelings places a stress upon the heart. But the real trap for the heart is a situation of lovelessness. Cousins said of himself that he felt love for his wife and children, but he questioned whether he had made it known and felt.

We don't know the intimate details of Cousins's personal life, and cardiologists generally don't probe into these matters when treating their patients. Statistics rarely help because the researchers do not ask the right questions. Such details are available, however, in psychotherapeutic case reports, and they often provide data that validate these concepts.

The patient who related the following was an internist who came for a consultation following his recovery from a heart attack. Ralph was a man in his late fifties who was in an unhappy second marriage. He had a daughter from his first marriage and two sons from the second. The trouble started early when, as Ralph said:

> I found that my second wife couldn't tolerate my daughter. She was like a witch, vindictive and vicious. Then she would be like a child. It was such a painful time. I tried to help her, but it didn't go. It was hell for me.
>
> About two years before the attack, I separated from my wife. But I couldn't stand the pain of a second divorce, this one involving my two sons, and I went back to her.
>
> About a year before the attack, I became desperate. I was impotent with my wife, so I decided to try other women—to shoot the works and have sex whenever and with whomever I felt like. I discovered that I wasn't impotent with other women, but these casual sexual affairs were not fulfilling. They had no relationship to my life.
>
> Then I fell in love with a younger woman named Mary who came to work as my nurse. One night I came home late from a date with her and found my wife very angry. In spite of her rage, I told her about this new relationship. But I couldn't stand up to her. She cowed me into renouncing Mary, which I wasn't ready to do, so I continued to see her on the sly.
>
> The day of the attack I had a drink with Mary before going home. That night my wife approached me sexually, and we made love. It was work. Although I had an ejaculation, I had no feeling of release, no sense of lightness afterward. I couldn't go to sleep. I felt a tightness just below the ribs. I went to the bathroom thinking that if I could move my bowels, it would

disappear. The pain seemed to subside, but when I went into the kitchen, it returned. It was a steady pain and seemed to increase. It lasted about ten minutes but was not a crushing pain. Still, I thought it could be a heart attack. My wife got out of bed, and I told her to take me to the hospital. On the way to the hospital I threw up several times involuntarily.

In the emergency room, I was hooked up to an EKG machine, but surprisingly, all the pain had disappeared. I felt disappointed that I had made the wrong diagnosis. But then the pain returned, and they gave me morphine. I fell asleep and while asleep suffered a cardiac arrest. The doctors restored the heartbeat, but I developed ventricular fibrillation, and they had difficulty stabilizing the rhythm. Waking up and watching the irregularity on the screen, I had a ghoulish sense of humor. I really didn't care if I lived or died. I didn't feel any panic. I had been embarrassed when I thought I had made a wrong diagnosis, and I was relieved that they had found it to be a heart attack. It was a posterior wall infarction.

I thought, Can I live long enough to survive this marriage? I felt the evening's sexual contact with my wife, the first since I had renounced Mary, was the final betrayal of myself.

Another heartbreaking thing had preceded the attack. Together with some associates, I had plans to build a clinic. Just before the heart attack, the venture became a financial disaster. I had to give up my dream and let go of my people. I felt defeated. I felt my wife had me by the balls.

We can learn much from this report, which clearly shows the powerful forces that engender a heart attack. The last remark indicates just how trapped Ralph felt in his marriage. But being in a trap cannot be regarded as the determining factor precipitating the attack. People have been trapped in unfulfilling marriages and other situations for years without anything dramatic happening. In my opinion, it is the sudden impulse to break out that when it collapses is the trigger. The collapse of the impulse leaves the person with a sense of hoplessness. One can tolerate being trapped in a painful situation as long as there is some hope in the heart. There is a saying that there is hope as long the heart beats. This implies that cardiac arrest is equivalent to a loss of hope. Ralph's heart attack was like a death knell and its occurrence must have been associated with a loss of hope. He did suffer a cardiac arrest.

How do hope and love fit together in our understanding of the heart? Isn't hope basically a hope for love, a hope for a meaningful and pleasurable connection to life, to the world about us, to someone or to some special individuals in that world? Life imprisonment isn't a death sentence if the prisoner makes such meaningful connection to his fellow inmates and to this particular world. But most life prisoners have some hope of release. We will discuss this aspect of the subject again in the next chapter. Our focus here is upon the role played by fear and panic in triggering the heart attack. Why couldn't Ralph get out of his marriage? What stopped him? (What frightened him?) I learned later that he eventually did divorce his wife. We must realize that the real trap is within, that the heart is imprisoned in a rigid cage and longs to be free to reach out for love. But to break out of this prison will evoke the pain of heartbreak and the fear of abandonment that can cause the person to panic and clamp down on the impulse. To squelch the impulse to reach out for love and freedom is, in effect, to clamp down on the heart, which can result in a spasm of one of the coronary arteries.

Spasm, in my opinion, is the key to an understanding of the heart attack. Coronary artery disease in the form of artheromatous plaques and thickening of the arterial wall predisposes the artery to an attack but is rarely in itself responsible for the total occulusion of the artery. Two observations support this view. People can suffer from severe coronary artery disease for some years without an attack occurring. And, on the other hand, a person can suffer a myocardial infarction without any previous history or coronary artery disease. We must ask, then, what causes the spasm. Spasms occur in muscular tissue other than that in the coronary artery. When a spasm hits a large striated muscle, we call it a cramp. We have all experienced such cramps in the muscles of the legs when we make a sudden, quick, or unusual movement. Such spasms do not occur in muscles that are fully relaxed or in muscles that are very contracted. In the latter case, no unusual movement is possible, while in the former case, all movements are free. An unusual movement occurs when a tense muscle begins to relax—that is, to move freely. The momentary loss of control provokes a reaction of fear in the tense muscle, which goes into spasm. Fortunately, such spasms or cramps are not dangerous and disappear with some relaxation. the situation is more serious when it happens in a coronary artery.

The victim of a heart attack is rarely conscious of this sequence of events. He may realize that he is trapped, but often he does not feel the overwhelming panic that the desire to break out arouses. This panic is the same panic he experienced in childhood in response to heartbreak, and just as he did then, he reacts to the threat his feelings pose by holding his breath and immobilizing his body on its deepest level, the heart.

Cousins's heart attack illustrates this sequence of events. As he relates, his attack occurred the day after he realized that he had no desire to go on yet another hectic business trip, despite the fact that he was scheduled to leave in a few days. His wish to withdraw from his obligations seems not to have been particularly strong, since he neither protested nor expressed anger at feeling trapped. Even when the attack occurred, he neither panicked nor cried out in pain. Instead, he accepted the situation in his typical good-humored way. But his equanimity was on the surface; inwardly, something had broken in his heart.

George Engel, a psychiatrist and internist, has written in some detail of the events preceding his own heart attack, which occurred nearly a year to the day after his twin brother, Frank, died of a heart attack at the age of forty-nine. His account sheds light on the role of unconscious guilt and hostility in precipitating a myocardial infarction.

The twins' own father had died of a heart attack two days before his fifty-ninth birthday. He died at home, leaving fifteen-year-old George, as he put it, with "pronounced feelings of unreality" and the conviction that he, like his father, would not reach his fifty-ninth birthday.

As children, Frank and George had been so alike that their parents had difficulty telling them apart. Their relationship, in George's words, was "close, intense but also extremely rivalrous." Both boys went to the same schools and pursued the same career. Frank became a professor of medicine and pathology at Duke University, and George became a professor of medicine and psychiatry at the University of Rochester.

Frank's death at forty-nine was entirely unexpected. Within hours after he heard of his brother's death, George experienced chest pain himself. A medical examination one week later revealed evidence of heart disease. Several of his dreams at the time were marked by confusion over whether he or his brother had died. George felt strongly that he might not live long after Frank's death. But as the months passed, George began to think that if he did not have an attack by July 10, the anniversary of Frank's death, then he would be spared. His own attack happened on July 9.

The day of the attack, George was scheduled to confront someone he closely identified with his brother. He did not look forward to the meeting and realized in retrospect that he had kept himself busy all week to avoid thinking about it. The meeting was scheduled for the evening of June 9. It never took place. At 3:30 in the afternoon, George had his heart attack.

"My reaction to the attack was great relief," he writes. "I felt serene and tranquil. Not only had I escaped the unpleasant meeting, but I no longer had to anticipate the attack."

This reaction may seem strange, but it occurs quite often, as we have noted, among heart attack victims. Clearly, the anxiety George felt about a possible attack was more stressful to him than the attack itself. Perhaps such underlying anxiety played a role in predisposing him to the attack, but his anxiety had other roots as well. These emerged as George listened to a radio performance of *Hamlet* while recovering from his attack.

> I suddenly thought I had achieved remarkable new insight into the play. Hamlet's uncle had not slain his brother. That was only Hamlet's fantasy. I was astonished that I had never appreciated this "fact" before, and I felt exhilarated at the discovery. Of course, I quickly realized my error and easily recognized its implications. I was not responsible for Frank's death at all!

George left the hospital, convalesced at home for a couple of months, and returned to a full load of work.

The reader may wonder how George could have felt responsible for his brother's death since there was no rational basis for such a thought. However, those familiar with psychoanalytic ideas will recognize that George's feeling of responsibility stemmed from an unconscious wish for Frank's death. As George admits, the sibling rivalry between the two brothers was intense. George recalls that he had once, in a fit of rage, chased his brother with a carving knife and had to be disarmed by the cook. As adolescents, they resolved never to date each other's girlfriend. No doubt such rivalry had its roots in infancy in the desire of each baby to have his mother fully to himself. Among animals, such rivalry is often a matter of survival when insufficient nurturing is available. Among humans it is more often a manifestation of sexual rivalry.

Like Norman Cousins, George Engel had difficulty handling negative feelings and suppressed them. In such instances, anxiety develops when these feelings move toward consciousness and the possibility of expression. This happened in George's case within the week preceding the anniversary of Frank's death.

One might say that George felt he had to be punished for wishing Frank's death.

In the years following his own coronary, George blocked out any further awareness of his feelings of guilt for his brother's death. However, on the fifth anniversary of Frank's death, he had an anxiety dream that he described as "the pain of guilt and loss over Frank's death and relief at my own survival." Another dream on the fifth anniversary of his own attack left him quite depressed, an emotional state he attributed to the conflict between his longing for reunion with his brother and the rivalry between them. Two other episodes in the ensuing years—the feeling that Frank had not died after all and a sudden attack of extreme fatigue that occurred exactly seven years to the minute after his own coronary—indicated that George was still struggling on an unconscious level.

George Engel calls his fear that he would not survive past fifty-eight, the age his father was when he died, his "nemesis complex." Such fears are also called "anniversary reactions." Olin, who has made a special study of anniversary reactions, describes them as "a psychobiologic response to the recollection at a specific time of a stressful event in the past destined to produce symptoms in the future . . . physical illness, such as heart attack; emotional illness, such as depression; and behavioral illness, such as substance abuse."[7] Olin refers to his own cases and also reports about some public figures. His story of Elvis Presley is especially relevant here. Presley was also a surviving twin and was very much involved with his dead brother. Moreover, as Olin reports, "Elvis and his mother were very attached. When she died, on August 14, 1958, at age 42, he said, 'My life has ended.' Nineteen years later, on August 6, 1977, he died at age 42."[8]

The year of nemesis for George Engel was his fifty-eighth year, his father's age at his death. During that year he thought more and more about his father, realizing how much he identified with him. In a photograph that his wife took of him at the time, George struck a pose so much like his father's that they could have been taken for twins. The fateful day his father had died was December 12, two days before his father's birthday and two days after George's own. In September, George began to have some ominous symptoms—progressive weakness, fatigue, breathlessness on exertion, and episodes of rapid heart action. He paid no attention until his physician, noticing his pallor, hospitalized him immediately. His symptoms proved to be anemia caused by the loss of a large amount of blood from bleeding hemorrhoids. The loss of blood was so great that it was life threatening. George had to receive a transfusion of two units of red blood cells, and it took him two weeks to recover. "But was it only that I was denying illness?" he asks. "Or could it be that I was passively accepting illness as a deserved fate, just as eight years earlier, I had passively accepted my heart attack?"[9]

Our interest in this case lies in the role critical anniversaries play in precipitating illness. Engel writes, "In this psychodynamic situation, calendar time in the form of anniversaries became the outside stimulus ever ready to reawaken the mortal life and death struggle."[10] For him, that struggle was between love and hate, first with his twin and then with his father for the love of his mother. But dare a boy be a bigger man than his father? To win against the father means to possess the mother, a crime that is beyond the pale.

We grow up and by some standards outperform our fathers, but the child within us, the forgotten child identified with the heart, stays the same. The split between the adult-ego aspect of our personality and the child-heart aspect fixates our deepest feelings at the level of a six-year-old at the end of the Oedipal phase. On that level, a boy cannot outdo his father; nor can he outlive him, for that, too, is a mark of superiority. For to be a better man than one's father means to possess the mother. In some cases this prospect is so terrifying that it seems to leave no alternative but to die.

The nemesis complex is more common in men than in women and is found mostly in relation to the father. Fortunately, it does not always end in death, though it may result in illness. In George's case, the threatened breakthrough of the unconscious hostility he felt toward his brother and his father ("I'm glad you're dead. Now I can have the field of glory all to myself") caused a panic reaction that ended in a spasm of the coronary arteries. In my opinion, every heart attack must be interpreted as a panic reaction on the unconscious level.

The panic reaction described above precedes the attack or is simultaneous with it. Once it occurs, the panic subsides, at least temporarily. It is amazing how few patients panic when they learn they have had a heart attack. In fact, many feel a sense of relief. Now the struggle is over.

One key to preventing heart attacks is to prevent panic. Norman Cousins is well aware of the dangers of panic for the heart, especially after an individual has suffered a coronary. "Panic intensifies underlying health problems," he writes. "Panic can contract the blood vessels, disrupt normal heart rhythms, and even cause myocardial infarction."[11] It is possible to deal with the panic that a person feels by reassuring him and making him feel less alone. But what are we to do for the panic-stricken person who feels no panic at all?

The first thing we must ask is how such a thing could be possible. We have seen that a split between body and mind allows feelings to occur on a physiological level without being perceived on a conscious level. Thus, a person may raise his shoulders, suck in his breath, and open his eyes wide—in other words, show all the signs of fear—without being aware that he is afraid. If the fear is deep and chronic, it extends into the interior organs and tissues. The smooth muscles of bronchi and arteries become spastic, the coronary arteries become rigid, and the stage is set for a heart attack following any acute response of fear or panic.

If a person can be made aware of the fear and panic he

harbors, he is less likely to experience a heart attack. Individuals who are subject to panic on the conscious level suffer emotionally, not physically, since as a general rule emotional illness precludes physical illness. There is abundant clinical evidence to support this observation. All psychiatrists have worked with patients who suffered from anxiety, often severe. In no case has such anxiety ever been reported to lead to a heart attack. I once treated a young man whose anxiety was so severe that it seriously handicapped his functioning and led him to contemplate suicide. He was aware that his anxiety was related in some way to a murderous rage he felt for his father but also toward me as a father substitute. At times it extended to other authority figures. His anxiety stemmed from the fear that his rage would erupt unexpectedly, with disastrous consequences. However, because he was aware of his rage, he was not a candidate for a heart attack.

In order to treat this problem, it is necessary to turn rage into anger, an emotion that can be integrated into the personality and handled rationally. But first the patient must vent his rage on a bed or other suitable object. He can whack the bed to his heart's content without feeling guilty that he is hurting someone. Then, once the pressure is released, he can begin to identify with his anger and express it appropriately in situations that call for an angry response.

Therapy aims at self-control, despite the fact that the patient is frequently encouraged to surrender to his feelings. There is nothing contradictory in this, since self-control implies the ability to surrender control in appropriate situations. For example, we should not let ourselves lose control when angry unless we are in a protected and controlled situation. On the other hand, we should not be afraid to surrender control in sex when we are expressing feelings of love. To develop healthy self-control, we need to be fully in touch with our feelings. The suppression of feeling undermines true self-control by splitting the unity of the personality. The denial of fear sets us up for the very thing we are afraid of. If we prevent ourselves from feeling heartbreak and deny our fear of aloneness, we make ourselves vulnerable to an attack that might literally break our hearts.

CHAPTER 8

Sudden Death

It has been estimated that about 450,000 cases of sudden death occur annually in the United States, accounting for 25 percent of the total.[1] According to De Silva and Lown, who have studied the phenomenon, "the typical victim, who is usually thought to be well prior to the event, is swiftly felled while engaging in his usual activities."[2] De Silva and Lown define such deaths as those "occurring instantaneously or within an estimated six hours after onset of acute symptoms and signs."[3] People tend to assume that a heart attack is the cause, but often an autopsy fails to reveal a myocardial infarction or the presence of a fresh coronary thrombosis (or clot) in one of the coronary arteries. However, the victim of sudden death is similar to other coronary artery patients in the prevalence of such risk factors as Type A behavior, hypertension, smoking, high cholesterol levels, and muscular rigidity associated with an inflated chest.

It is now generally recognized that the process of ventricular fibrillation is the "terminal mechanism"[4] of sudden death in almost every case. Ventricular fibrillation is defined as "a chaotic electrical depolarization of the heart resulting in disorganized and ineffective mechanical activity with cessation of blood flow."[5] Because the heartbeat is very chaotic and rapid, the heart is unable to propel the blood. Death occurs in minutes if cardiopulmonary resuscitation and defibrillation are not applied.

The question we shall attempt to answer here is what happens to cause a heart that is beating normally to develop a fatal arrhythmia, or abnormal rhythm. At the outset we must recognize that a healthy heart does not beat like a clock. As we know, the heart rate speeds up or slows down in response to the needs of the body for blood. Thus, when a person is engaged in strenuous physical activity, the heart rate may go up from a resting rate of 70 beats per minute to as many as 130 beats. In a state of ease and relaxation, the heart rate slows down. But physical activity is not the only cause of a more rapid heartbeat. All emotional states directly affect the heart. Love as well as fear can cause the heart to beat faster. Such reactions are not arrhythmias but variations in the normal rhythm. They are not, therefore, pathological.

Skipping an occasional heartbeat is a common form of arrhythmia. Probably everyone has experienced it, since it can happen to a perfectly normal heart. However, the heart does not skip a beat by chance. A flutter of the heart denotes anxiety in just the same way as butterflies in the belly. In the case of a single missed beat, the anxiety may be so minor that it escapes awareness. On the other hand, when the heart starts to flutter, it is almost impossible not to feel anxious.

In normal circumstances, the heartbeat is a wave of contraction that spreads through the heart muscle in an orderly way. It is preceded by certain electrical phenomena that trigger the contraction of the individual muscle cells. An electrocardiogram picks up the electrical component of this wave and lets us know if there is any disturbance in its flow. But to speak of electrical instability as a cause of sudden death is to think of the heart in purely mechanical terms. Neither a person nor his heart is an electrical system, although there is an electrical aspect to the body's functioning.

My thesis is that an unstable heart exists in an unstable person. Emotions are the life of the body. An open and loving heart exists in a loving person; a cold and closed heart, in an indifferent person. Instability of any kind denotes a disturbance in the whole personality.

The operation of the defibrillator demonstrates the emotional key to ventricular fibrillation, panic. The defibrillator is an apparatus that uses an electrical current to apply a shock to the heart. Like the hard slap that snaps a panic-stricken individual back to reality, the shock stops all cardiac activity momentarily, which serves in most instances to restore the heart's rhythm. In rate instances, two or more shocks must be applied to restore normal rhythm.

In many cases, a direct connection exists between panic and sudden death. Individuals confronted by fires or other natural catastrophes have been known to panic and to die of heart attacks. Their hearts may have been less stable in the first place, but the individuals themselves may have been less stable emotionally than those who remained calm and survived the event.

Panic represents the struggle against a sense of being trapped in a life-threatening situation. If the organism gives up the struggle and accepts its fate, the panic disappears. Experimental evidence derived from animal studies strongly supports this view. In one study reported by De Silva and Lown, dogs were exposed to electric shocks they could not avoid. Although the dogs had perfectly normal hearts, they showed a more than 40 percent increase in vulnerability to ventricular fibrillation. Their heart rates increased, as did their blood pressure and the level of "struggle hormones" in their blood. All these physiological changes denoted heightened activity in the sympathetic nervous system, that part of the autonomic nervous system that prepares an animal for fight or flight. In those dogs whose hearts had been previously damaged by blocked coronary arteries, the shock conditioning evoked ventricular fibrillation.

Researchers found that these effects could be nullified by procedures that blocked the sympathetic system. Drugs such as propranolol and tolamolol, which are inhibitors of sympathetic action, protected those animals undergoing coronary artery occlusion against ventricular fibrillation. Cutting the sympathetic nerves to the heart had a similar effect. And morphine, which diminishes pain, provided significant protection against fibrillation in conscious animals undergoing stress. All of these procedures had the effect of reducing or preventing the fear reaction.[6]

The following case report of a fourteen-year-old girl who lost consciousness when she was awakened one night by a thunderclap shows dramatically the role of fear in producing ventricular fibrillation. After that experience, whenever the girl was awakened by the ring of an alarm clock, the fall of a large object, or another loud sound, she would go into an episode of ventricular fibrillation and lose consciousness. These episodes were short and self-terminating, and careful examination failed to reveal any heart abnormality.[7] It was assumed that an electrically unstable heart predisposed her to these episodes. Unfortunately, no in-depth psychological study of the girl was done to determine her emotional state. Was she a frightened person? Did she suffer from nightmares? Had she experienced any emotional trauma in her childhood?

Lown reports an unusual case in which fear was implicated in the sudden death of a thirty-nine-year-old man whose heart was structurally normal. Ventricular fibrillation occurred during early-morning sleep while the man was under study at a sleep clinic. He had entered the clinic complaining that he usually experienced dreams with a violent content at this time. At his death, the electrocephalogram to which he was routinely attached confirmed that severe heartbeat irregularities had coincided with his REM (or deep) sleep.[8]

In *The Healing Heart*, Norman Cousins calls panic "the ultimate enemy,"[9] particularly the panic patients feel when they learn that they have a serious illness. He says (and I agree) that "nothing is more essential in the treatment of serious disease than liberating the patient from panic and foreboding."[10] The "sudden catecholamine [epinephrine] flooding [which occurs in panic] can precipitate a wide range of negative reactions, not excluding cardiac destabilization and constriction of blood vessels."[11] Anything that can allay panic—such as human contact, support, and reassurance—is helpful. Cousins's particular antidote is laughter, which he has found useful in his own life as well as in his work with patients. Like crying, laughing promotes respiration, providing the body and the heart with needed oxygen.

Cousins recounts a case that shows graphically the destructive effect of panic on the heart's functioning. The case involved a young man who took a cardiogram as part of a regular physical examination. To his utter surprise, the cardiogram revealed evidence of a previous heart attack. The young man, who thought he was in excellent health, denied any knowledge of such an event. That night, however, he developed chest pains for the first time and panicked. The next three days were a nightmare. He lost seventeen pounds and was tormented by thoughts of death. A stress test revealed cardiac weakness, and an angiogram showed a lesion in one of the coronary arteries. Bypass surgery was recommended.

Cousins relates how he helped the young man overcome his panic by assuring him that with confidence and practice his heart would perform well. On a subsequent stress test, the young man showed no evidence of cardiac or respiratory difficulty. Six months later, after observing a sensible life-style and a program of proper health care, a second angiogram revealed no trace of the lesion. The young man never had the bypass.

This case is interesting not only as an example of the heart's capacity to heal itself when emotional stresses are reduced or eliminated but also as an illustration of the fact that panic, when expressed, does not kill. This man lived in a state of continuous panic for three days without developing ventricular fibrillation. His conscious experience of panic may have affected his whole body, but it spared his heart. I have emphasized throughout this study that it is the suppression of feeling that produces somatic illness.

I myself encountered a case of sudden cardiac arrest in which the suppression of feeling was fairly evident. The victim was a former patient of mine called Benjamin, and the precipitating event, I learned later from his wife, was the unwelcome prospect of retirement. More heart attacks are associated with retirement than with any other event.

Benjamin had been in treatment with me some thirty years earlier, and I had kept in touch with him over the years. No one would ever have described him as a Type A individual. He was neither competitive nor aggressive, neither pressured to achieve nor laboring under a sense of time urgency. Nor did he suffer from a lack of self-esteem. Instead, he felt superior, a feeling based on a generous nature, a sensitivity to people, and an educated mind. He was self-taught, but his education had been thorough. Yet I knew that underneath his facade he lacked self-confidence and tended toward passivity. He was sixty-six years old and on the verge of retiring from his job as a foreman in a machine shop when he died suddenly.

It happened as follows: One weekday morning a friend called for Benjamin in his car to take him to the train station. On the way, Benjamin just keeled over. His friend drove him home and called for an ambulance. He also went for Benjamin's wife, who arrived home to find Benjamin sprawled on the grass with the paramedics working to resuscitate him. Their efforts were unsuccessful. An autopsy determined that the cause of death was ventricular fibrillation with underlying coronary atherosclerosis.

Benjamin had no history of heart disease and had never complained of angina or chest pains. He smoked cigarettes and led a sedentary life, but he was not overweight. Knowing him as well as I did, I knew that he had considerable suppressed anger. He was vulnerable to heart disease, but that didn't explain his sudden death. What happened to Benjamin to cause this fearful event? His wife provided some information about his emotional state at the time of his death. "The day before he died," she said, "I told him to go to management and tell them he was retiring the first of the year. He had been saying for some time that he was going to retire, but he also said that he was going to work until the day he died. He did. He was ambivalent about retiring."

Retirement for Benjamin meant moving to another city where it was cheaper to live. He and his wife had already put down a deposit on a new house. "About two or three weeks before he died," his wife told me, "he visited some friends who knew about this planned move. They told me that he had said to them, 'But I'll never live in that house. I'll die.' He died before the closing."

Benjamin had become deeply religious during the past several years. Moving to another city would have forced him to break off a very close relationship with the minister of the church in which he was a deacon. At the same time, his relationship with his wife had deteriorated. Their sexual life had dropped off almost to nothing during this period.

Had Benjamin been more secure in his relationship with his wife, the prospect of retirement might not have been so frightening. But he was afraid of his wife, just as he was afraid, to some degree, of all women. As a child, his mother had tied him to her in a way that prevented him from identifying fully with his father. She had restricted his aggression while encouraging him to develop his sensitive side. Close as he was to his mother, his natural sexual interest in her was taboo. He did not feel connected to her by love; even at the time of his death, she possessed him, and he was afraid of her. Nor did he feel connected to his wife. His real connections were outside the home—to his fellow workers, the men who shared his musical interests, and the church. The prospect of giving them up and finding himself tied to a woman was too frightening to bear. He knew he couldn't do it, and yet he couldn't say no. Unable to flee or fight, he was trapped. I believe that the panic evoked by this situation killed him.

The case of Carl, a sixty-year-old sportswriter, also illustrates the trauma of retirement. Carl was an avid tennis player and in good physical shape. However, he faced mandatory retirement at the age of sixty. He accepted it with dignity, but he also felt considerable anger and resentment toward his employers. He did not express these feelings, but they were reflected in his dreams. For several months after retirement, he had a recurrent dream of being needed. Other dreams were full of longing and deep sadness. One morning he collapsed and was rushed to the hospital, where his life was saved by prompt treatment with a defibrillator.

The story of Paul William "Bear" Bryant, the "winningest coach" in college football, ended less happily. Shortly after his retirement, he died suddenly and unexpectedly of a massive heart attack. It was widely said that he died of a broken heart. Football was the life he loved, and when he gave it up, he severed his most vital connection.

When death is caused by ventricular fibrillation, we are justified in describing it as a panic reaction. However, cardiac arrest can occur without ventricular fibrillation, perhaps because some people are able to accept death calmly. Engel describes a case reported in *Life* magazine in which there was no indication of panic. The man described in the article was in his seventies. Independent and unmarried, he had made complete preparations for his death and burial, even to the point of supervising the landscaping of his burial plot. He seemed to all who knew him to be in good spirits. One week after a medical examination showed him to be in good health, he gathered his family together and, over their protests, distributed his property, saying, "I don't need anything anymore." Engel relates that "as the last item was disposed of, he dropped dead before his astonished relatives."[12]

When death comes naturally at the end of a full life, a person goes to sleep quietly, but it is a sleep with no awakening. Such deaths are common in the animal kingdom but relatively rare among civilized people, for whom there is often a struggle between a wish to die and the will to live. Primitive peoples, on the other hand, are better able to allow themselves to die without struggle or conflict, especially in the case of so-called voodoo deaths. Several investigators have studied this phenomenon.[13] Voodoo death has been reported among the natives of South America, Africa, Australia, New Zealand, Haiti, and the islands of the Pacific. As one observer noted, "I saw an old woman cast a spell on a man. 'You will die before sunset,' she told him. And he did. At autopsy, no cause of death could be found."[14]

When a curse is laid upon a primitive, it is assumed he has been possessed by evil spirits, and he is ostracized by the community. In effect, all his connections to the community, including members of his family, are severed. Without these, he is a nonentity, with no right to life. He may not choose to die, but he has no alternative. Without vital connections, life cannot go on. Without love, the heart stops.

As civilized people, we may feel ourselves to be less vulnerable to such beliefs, but in fact they simply take different forms, as we saw in this chapter. George Engel felt cursed by his father's and his brother's deaths. Benjamin felt cursed by the prospect of retirement. J. J. Mathis reports the case of a fifty-three-year-old man who died suddenly in an acute asthmatic attack within an hour of defying his mother's prediction of "dire consequences" if he acted against her wishes.[15]

Children are especially vulnerable to maledictions from someone they regard as powerful. If a mother says to her young child, "No one will ever love you; you are impossible," he is likely to believe her. As he grows up and his ego and rational mind assume control of his behavior, he may see himself as worthy of love despite his mother's curse, but deep in his heart he will always wonder if she was right. Moreover, because he feels required to earn love by his own efforts, he will always feel some degree of isolation.

Nothing is more frightening to a child than the feeling of being lost and alone in the world. That fear may diminish in adults, but it never completely disappears. No animal experiences its aloneness in quite the same way, for it feels itself to be part of the larger order of nature. Man's fear stems from his self-consciousness and from the fact that he is the most helpless and dependent of creatures at birth. An extended period of motherly love is the key to human survival. As we shall see in the next chapter, the loss of love is so powerful and threatening that those who suffer it experience a wish to die.

CHAPTER 9

The Will to Live and the Wish to Die

Self-destructive behavior is one of the most difficult phenomena to comprehend. Such behavior is relatively rare in animals but fairly common in humans. People who drink, take drugs, smoke, or overeat know on some level that their behavior is harmful. I knew one person who described each cigarette as a coffin nail, but he could not control his habit; eventually, he died from cancer. The idea that he wished to die cannot be dismissed but it is not the whole story. Also operating in such people, albeit unconsciously, is suppressed anger. Suicide is the best example of this. Most psychologists recognize that the impulse to kill one's self has at its core a desire to kill someone else: a parent, spouse, or former lover. The suppression of this desire out of guilt turns the murderous impulse against the self.

Since suppressed anger and hostility are characteristic of Type A behavior, it should come as no surprise that Type A individuals show marked self-destructive tendencies. Friedman describes two successful chief executives who failed to file income tax returns, an "oversight" that cost them their careers.[1] Did these men, otherwise healthy and seemingly normal, want to be caught? Does the Type A man who suffers a heart attack want to fall ill? Surprisingly, some admit to such feelings. Friedman learned that over half of the men in his study who had incurred an infarction not only expected to have an attack but yearned for it. "It's so damned nice to lie here and have no resonsibilities and to have such pretty nurses taking good care of me," said one of them. Said another: "Now I can retire from the company and begin to live like a real human being again. You know what? I wanted this to happen, and I didn't care whether I lived or not."

For some people, a heart attack may seem the only way to escape the stresses and strains of a pressured existence. Some then go on to make the kind of changes in their lives that might have prevented the attack. Is there in such people a need to suffer, stemming perhaps from some deep sense of guilt, so that only after they have paid a price are they free to make some positive moves in their lives? There is no question but that self-destructive tendencies can have a powerful grip on the personality so that the individual feels literally trapped and unable to deal with his life. Since the forces that motivate such behavior are internal and largely unconscious, they are resistant to the conscious will. But until they are understood and their origin explained, they render the conscious will impotent.

Psychiatrists are aware that illness often provides secondary rewards or gains to the patient. The ill person receives a degree of care and concern that he may never have experienced before and is catered to like an infant with no responsibilities. Some illness can be seen as an emotional unconscious regression, an attempt to gain the love one didn't get as an infant. But in fact the sick person is not loved unconditionally, since the care is extended because of his illness, and the caretaker inevitably feels some resentment at the burden sickness places on the healthy. (I am not speaking of doctors and nurses, who accept this burden in their personal choice of profession, but of family members, who are themselves struggling to be free.) If illness is the price of such attention, it is inordinately high. Moreover, a heart attack poses an immediate threat to life with no guarantee of survival, so it is not just a question of wishing to be ill to gain attention or care but of wishing to die.

Individuals often express a wish to die; some act upon it. Those with suicidal thoughts have a conscious wish to die, which they actually attribute to the painfulness and hopelessness of their lives. A suicidal thought or fantasy represents the feeling "I can't stand it any longer." But suicide has another meaning, too. Ordinarily, if a person can't stand a situation, he tries to change it. But the suicidal person believes change is impossible because what he wants to change is the behavior of others toward him. He wants the unconditional acceptance and love that he didn't get as a child from his parents and that he feels he needs. When it is not forthcoming, he feels deprived and full of rage. This rage is further fueled by the feeling that others have expectations of him that he cannot satisfy. At the same time, he harbors a great sense of guilt about his anger. Because he feels inadequate and unlovable, he turns his anger against himself. In destroying himself, he is also trying to hurt others. He is convinced they will suffer, and sometimes they do.

A divorced woman in her forties with two children was involved in a love relationship with a man who said he couldn't marry her as long as his mother was alive. The woman believed him despite the efforts of friends to make her see that his explanation was only an excuse. The relationship went on for a number of years, and his mother finally died. But when the woman pressed her lover to marry her, he broke off the relationship. She then tried twice to commit suicide in an attempt to make the man feel guilty about his behavior. When her attempts failed to have this effect, she tried a third time to kill herself, and succeeded.

Such self-destructive behavior, taken to the nth degree, clearly stems from the denial of anger. Suppressed anger is like holding a knife to one's breast. But what keeps the anger suppressed? In other words, what is the basis for self-destructive behavior? If we answer fear, we must ask: fear of what and of whom? The person who suppresses his anger is not aware that he does so out of fear. In most cases, the fear is equally suppressed, and the person has no clear memory of early situations in which he felt both angry and afraid—in particular, afraid that he would be punished for his anger. Not until he is able to remember and reexperience some of these feelings can we fully understand why he is driven to self-destructive behavior. This process generally takes place in an analytic program, the primary aim of which is to help him understand and change such behavior.

As Freud recognized early on, every analytic therapy is characterized by resistance and transference. Resistance refers to an unconscious blocking of the therapist's efforts to help the patient get in touch with his early life, despite the patient's awareness that his recovery depends on the insights he gains from making connections to his past. Transference refers to the patient's behavior vis-à-vis the therapist. Since he is in a subordinate position and needs help, he sees the therapist as a substitute parent toward whom he transfers or projects the conflicting feelings he felt toward his real parent. At the same time that he expects the therapist to take care of him as a good parent should, he sees the therapist as a bad parent who will take advantage of his need for his own benefit. In most cases, the patient conceals his distrust and negative feelings about the therapist, fearful that if he expresses them, the therapist will become angry and refuse to help him. Because it impedes the therapeutic process, holding back negative thoughts is another form of resistance.

As a result of the transference, the patient recreates in the analytic relationship the same situation that produced his neurosis. This process gives the analyst or therapist a chance to understand how the neurosis arose in the first place. Theoretically, analysis of the transference should free the patient from his fixation in that early situation. It rarely does, however, because the patient's unconscious resistance to revealing all his thoughts and feelings make the analysis of the transference difficult to complete. The patient is trapped in his transference, and the therapist is trapped equally in his countertransference (in other words, his need to help). Analytic or therapeutic failure is therefore quite common. The patient continues to repeat his neurotic behavior despite its evident self-destructive nature. Witnessing this behavior time and again, Freud called it the repetition compulsion—the compulsion patients have to reenact the same traumatic and disappointing scenario throughout their lives.

Confronted with the phenomena of resistance, transference, and the repetition compulsion, Freud postulated the existence of a death instinct, called Thanatos, to explain self-destructive behavior. As a counterbalance to the destructive effects of the death instinct, Freud invoked the idea of a life instinct called Eros. In the healthy individual, he theorized, Eros directs the death instinct away from the self and out into the world as anger or aggression. However, if the life instinct is not strong enough to do this and the personality is dominated by the death instinct, anger is turned inward against the self, creating a condition Freud called masochism.

Many analysts have accepted such notions, but I, for one, have never been able to accept the concept of a death instinct. The word *instinct* has always been associated in my mind with life. We cannot deny, however, that some people drive themselves to death. In their case, it would seem the life forces aren't strong enough to prevent self-destructive behavior. But this doesn't mean that such behavior is natural or instinctive. We must look more deeply into the personality and more closely at the events of early life to understand how such self-destructive forces develop.

"If I breathe, I will die," a patient of mine said. Breathing is certainly not self-destructive. Quite the contrary, holding one's breath is anti-life. How, then, could the patient associate breathing with death?

The answer to this question holds the key to an understanding of resistance and therefore of the tendency to self-destructive behavior. The deeper and fuller a person breathes, the more alive he is. The more alive he is, the more he feels. But when his feelings are so painful that they are unbearable, he will do everything possible not to make contact with them, namely, to resist and deny that he has such feelings and to breathe shallowly so as not to feel them.

This is the same patient whose case I had reported earlier. Her mother had let her cry for so long as a baby that she had vomited and nearly choked to death. That experience had left an indelible impression on the young organism: to want love desperately is to risk a painful death. One traumatic incident may not seriously handicap a child but, in this as in most cases, it may represent a pattern in the relationship of parent to child. The amazing part of this story is that my patient heard it from her mother, who related it with pride. She had not given in to the child. She saw the incident as a power struggle with the child that she had won. The child, meanwhile, had lost—not the power struggle, for it is impossible to conceive that a two-month-old baby has any idea of power, but any faith she had in her mother. While mother and daughter seemed to get along after the incident, theirs was no longer a heart-to-heart relationship. As a result, the patient suffered from depression most of her adult life. She had to push herself to perform her daily activities and said that if she stopped pushing, if she just lay down, she would not get up again. This feeling reflects the person's struggle to survive despite the heartbreaking pain of the loss of love. Since life is meaningless without love, survival requires a great effort of will to overcome the desire to give up and die.

Most people who have suffered the loss of love counter this

wish to die by not giving up, by continuing the struggle to earn love by achieving, by serving, and by trying to fulfill other people's expectations. They *must* succeed; they *will* succeed. Their jaws are set in a grim determination not to fail, for failure means death. Instead, they mobilize a conscious *will to live*. The will declares: "I won't break down, I'll keep going on, I won't need you." Used to suppress feelings, the will is the source of resistance in therapy and a major obstacle to health.

How common is the wish to die? I have heard many patients express it, and I have learned to take it seriously after one patient committed suicide. I don't regard every patient who utters these words as a potential suicide, but every time I hear them, I am keenly aware of the depth and amount of pain in the personality. I also know that the person doesn't want to die, that he has a wish to live. The two wishes, one to live and one to die, can coexist because they come from different layers of the personality. In evaluating the possibility of suicide, it is necessary to weigh the strength of each of these feelings.

I don't believe I would have known how widespread the wish to die was until I experienced it myself. Some years ago while I was swimming slowly and easily in a pool, the thought crossed my mind as my head was under water that I didn't want to lift it up again. To lift up my head required making an effort, and I was tired of making efforts. How nice just to lie there and do nothing. It would be like a return to the womb. But I knew that if I didn't lift my head out of the water to breathe, I would die. The thought was not particularly frightening, but I sensed that I wanted to live. I lifted my head up, breathed in, and continued swimming, but the experience left me with an awareness of how much of a struggle life was for me.

As I work with my patients, I see that for all of them life is a struggle, for some a grim one, which leaves little room for real pleasure and enjoyment. But they are not unique. For almost all of us life has this quality. So many of us are deeply tired of the endless struggle of our lives. Yet if we are to recover the feeling of joy in life, we must give up the struggle. For adults, the war is over. We lost, and we can no longer get the unconditional love from our parents that we needed and so desperately wanted as children. We waste our energies continuously struggling for it. To accept the loss is painful and an admission of failure, which the ego fights against, but acceptance liberates us from our involvement with the past. Only by accepting the past are we free to move toward a more fulfilling future.[2] As proof of this, I point out to my patients that the two nations who lost the Second World War are now the most successful nations on earth.

On a deep, unconscious level, a patient fears that to give up or surrender the will is to die. Since he has survived by the use of the will, letting go of the will and giving in to his feelings might end in death. Of course, such an outcome isn't likely because most patients wish to live. When one gets a person to feel the desire to live, self-destructive behavior diminishes or ends.

Therapy aims at helping a person make direct contact with his life force so that he can draw on it for his own fulfillment. But to make this contact, he must dig below the first two layers of his personality, namely the will to live and the wish to die. Figure 13 illustrates this layering. The will to live derives its energy from the life force by drawing energy from the aim of fulfillment to that of survival.

The first step for the patient is to become aware of the conflict between his will to live and his wish to die. That awareness can sometimes be achieved through a bioenergetic exercise. In one such exercise, the person lies over a bioenergetic stool and breathes out as deeply as possible. At the end of the expiration, he is instructed not to breathe in. How the patient handles this situation provides some insight into his personality. When he has to breathe in right after a relatively short expiration, it is evidence of the presence of panic. Many patients experience this panic, which they explain by saying, "I need

Figure 13. The will to live and the wish to die

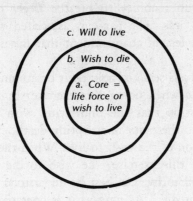

a. The word core is derived from the Latin root cor,
which means heart. The French word coeur and the Span-
ish word corazon reflect this identity. The heart is at the
core of life. Feeling the heart connects one strongly with
the wish to live.
b. The wish to die is the layer that contains the pain, the
sadness, and the despair at the loss of love. It is the layer
of heartbreak.
c. The will to live is the ego's survival technique. Based
on building defenses against pain, sadness, and despair,
it blocks the heart's desire to reach out for love.

air," or "I feel that if I don't breathe in, I'll die." But it is
impossible to die from a deliberate effort not to breathe. When
the need for air is acute, the body will take over and breathe
against any conscious effort to restrain it.

We know that the breath can be held for fairly long periods
of time. Anyone who has done underwater swimming without a
tank knows that the breath can be held for some minutes. I
believe that ten minutes is the record with a person lying still
under water. However, holding the breath in is not what our
exercise accomplishes. Underwater swimmers hold the air *in*
after a deep *inspiration*. In the above exercise, air is held *out* after
a deep *expiration*. Because the body normally has a two- to
three-minute reserve supply of oxygen in the lungs and blood,

the panic the patient feels is not the result of a lack of air or oxygen but of an inability to breathe freely due to chronic tension in the chest. The panic is associated with a sense of insecurity and a fear of abandonment that raises the specter of death.

Other individuals seem to hold their breath out for an inordinately long time when doing this exercise. In their case, one gets the impression that the underlying wish to die is very strong, almost to the point of accepting death, since to breathe in is an expression of the wish to live. When the will to live is immobilized by this exercise, the wish to die becomes more evident. The will to live can best be understood in its negative form: "I will not die." As long as it is operative, the person's breathing is fairly regular but shallow; the will keeps respiration at a level where deep feelings such as despair are not touched. By getting the person to breathe deeply, especially on expiration, the will's defensive function is bypassed, allowing the person to come closer to the feeling of despair and the wish to die. This explains the panic in the first group, those who are afraid to let the air out fully. They, too, have a wish to die, which frightens them greatly, but it is countered by a strong will to live. In the second group, the will to live is weaker.

There is also a group of people in the middle whose will is not strongly engaged because the wish to die is weak or absent. This group can breathe out deeply and hold the air out long enough to excite a powerful gasp. Such a gasp is a spontaneous, life-affirming action identical in every way to the first cry and breath of a newborn infant. The intensity with which air is sucked into the body is a measure of the strength of the wish to live. In gasping, the throat opens wide to take in as much air as possible, which is tantamount to opening fully to life. After the gasp the person breathes more deeply and fully and frequently breaks into soft, deep sobs. Such crying is an expression of relief—that one need not resist life because of a fear of death or a fear of feeling.

The wish to live is the psychological side of the biological instinct for self-preservation. It is at the core of the personality and is manifested in all life-maintaining functions of the body: the beating of the heart, the peristaltic waves of the intestines, the expansion and contraction of respiration, plus all the myriad activities of the different organs, tissues, and cells. Breathing is the most visible of these functions and can serve, therefore, as an indication of the strength of the life force. How deeply a person breathes reflects the strength of his wish to live. Does the wave of inspiration extend down into the abdomen to reach the pelvic floor? Is breathing a total bodily activity, or is it limited to one segment, the chest or the diaphragm? The opposite of deep breathing is shallow, restricted, or forced breathing. It is not a question of how much air one can take in with effort but how much air one takes in without effort. Since *breathing in* is a process of sucking in the air, we are also measuring the strength of the sucking impulse. Any childhood experiences that have weakened the strength of this impulse have also reduced the strength of the desire to live. Any exercise such as the one described above that mobilizes and strengthens this impulse will increase the person's energy and desire to live. If crying can be evoked, it will diminish the stress on the heart and greatly stimulate breathing by reducing the muscular tensions and rigidities that handicap the basic life-promoting actions of the body.

People characterized by a strong will to live can be called survivors, a term that applies to so many individuals in our culture. Their bodies are marked by tight jaws and overall rigidity. Despite their apparent ability to survive, they remain at the level of pain and despair associated with their original loss of love, which led in the first place to the wish to die. This wish is constantly reinforced by the lack of fulfillment (love) that goes hand in hand with the individual's preoccupation with survival. Living on an emergency basis, albeit unconsciously, they are poised for fight or flight, but do neither. Their rigidity allows them to hold on and to survive, but they cannot find fulfillment. And because of the enormous stress on the body, holding on cannot be assured indefinitely, which threatens their very survival. Sooner or later they become exhausted and wish to give up. At this point they may panic (in other words, feel the wish to die) and experience a heart attack.

To avoid such an outcome, a person must surrender his will and freely experience his pain, despair, and wish to die so that he can mourn the loss of love and grieve for the years he struggled. Such a surrender allows him to contact his life force at its very core: the impulse to breathe and the wish to live. Love is the heart of life, and the heart is the source of love. One must penetrate to the core of one's being to find the love that is the meaning and fulfillment of life.

A good example of this process can be seen in the following report of a therapeutic session at a training workshop with a young man, a clinical psychologist who had come to study bioenergetic analysis. At the lunch break, he decided to try the bioenergetic stool. As he was lying over the stool, I happened to pass by and saw a look of death on his face. I remarked on this to him, so after lunch he volunteered to work with me. Standing before the group, he said, "I was surprised by your observation. I have been preoccupied with death lately. My wife committed suicide about three months ago." But the expression on his face had a chronic quality. Furthermore, a tense jaw betrayed a strong will to live to balance a wish to die.

I suggested that he try the exercise described above. He was willing. It generally takes several attempts at holding the air out before a patient can muster the courage to stay without inhaling long enough to mobilize a powerful gasp. That was the case with this patient. Then the throat opened, and the gasp broke through. He began to sob deeply, "I want to live, I want to live," he kept saying.

After the exercise, I asked him if he had ever come close to death. "Yes," he said, "I almost died when I was a baby. In fact, the doctors didn't expect me to live. I wouldn't eat and kept losing weight."

I asked him what had happened at that time in his life. He said, "My mother weaned me."

The patient's set jaw expressed his determination not to reach out to his mother's breast with his mouth because the frustration was too painful. At the same time, it also expressed his determination to survive without the love he wanted. By not opening up and reaching out, he could avoid the pain of rejection. But living on a survival level kept him involved in a life-and-death struggle that showed on his face.

I proposed that he try to discharge the pain of the past, which fed his wish to die, by reaching out to his mother now, thereby evoking the pain of that early trauma. No longer a child, he could accept the pain rather than fight it. He lay on the couch and extended his lips, reaching up with his arms at the same time and calling for his mother. I applied a steady pressure to the tight muscles of his jaw. He then broke into such heartrending sobs that all of us present in the room could feel the agony of the baby (still present in the adult) at the loss of his world, the breast of the mother, which represented joy and fulfillment. Psychologically, the baby had no wish to die, but the pain of the loss was so great that the baby's throat contracted to the point that eating was almost impossible.

When the exercise was over, the patient said that he felt much freer than before. He had known the story of his illness but had never connected it with the loss of the breast. I am sure that his mother and his doctors had failed to make that connection, too. As a result, the baby was left in an extremely hopeless and helpless position that crying couldn't seem to remedy. The crying the patient did now, coupled with an understanding of his loss, washed the look of death and pain from his face.

Not every case is as dramatic as this one. In many it is not easy for the patient to get past the will to live and experience the wish to die. One often hears the words, "I want to die," but the fear of death is too strong to permit a confrontation. One has to work with some patients for a long time before they gain the courage to experience it. One can assure the patient that he will not die in this confrontation. He survived the real experience when he was younger and helpless, and now he also has the therapist's support.

When a person dies, his death can be seen as an expression of a biological wish to die. On a psychological level, he may still feel the will to live, which represents the position of the ego or conscious mind and not necessarily the wishes of the body. It can be said, therefore, that when a person dies from natural causes he lived as long as *he wished.* The will to live is effective only so long as it is energized by the life force of the organism. The collapse of this life force from exhaustion or stress undermines the will to live.

It has been found in several studies that cancer often develops in older people following the loss of a loved one. It is assumed, and rightly so, that the stress of the loss produces the illness. Many researchers have recognized, however, that this loss in later life repeats a similar trauma in childhood, namely, the loss of the love of a mother or father. The later loss activates the pain of the earlier one, increasing the wish to die. In many cases, the wish to die is conscious, for with advanced age there is a sense of hopelessness about finding new love. Without love or the hope for love, one cannot even survive.

We began this chapter with a discussion of the self-destructive behavior of cardiac patients. The most common form is the behavior of the Type A individual, who is driven to achieve, to prove he is worthy of love. The intensity of that drive reveals its desperate quality. One patient put it this way: Life is such a struggle. If I give up the struggle, I give up life. I don't know how to live for me. I am involved in raising my family, getting my children married, working, etc. All my life has been a continual effort to justify my existence because I wasn't supposed to be there. My mother didn't want another child, but if there was to be one, she wanted a girl. When I was born, she said, "Take him away. He's not mine." It is impossible to know why his mother told him this story, which placed a terrible burden upon him.

Many readers are familiar with Norman Cousins's book about his first major illness, *The Anatomy of an Illness*. That illness proved to be a collagen disease that came on suddenly and was nearly fatal. Cousins attributes his cure to a regimen of laughter and vitamin C, both in very high doses. His account of the events just prior to the onset of the illness reveals that he experienced an extreme degree of fatigue resulting from stress. But he could not accept the exhaustion because his will demanded that he carry on. Illness develops when a person pushes himself beyond the breaking point. Unfortunately, he does not always recognize the breaking point until he has passed it. The danger is not in the state of exhaustion itself but in the belief, conscious or unconscious, that to give in to tiredness is a sign of weakness, that it is unacceptable to say, "I can't."

Quite the opposite is true. Giving in to one's tiredness allows a person to convalesce, to renew his energy and recover his spirit. Giving in to one's sadness opens and releases the deep pain of heartbreak. That pain resides in the body: in the tight jaw, constricted throat, rigidly held chest, and sucked-in belly of the person who suppresses his longing for love and his wish to live.

Having closed off the longing for love, the person no longer feels the pain. To the degree that he is closed off, all he can feel is a deep sense of frustration and hopelessness that fuels the wish to die. To reach out, on the other hand, makes the pain come alive. There is no pain in death, which is the great appeal of death for so many people. There is no pain in life, either, if one is fully alive. Then the flow of feeling is free and unrestricted. The pain is in coming alive, in the flow of energy and feeling into tight or dead areas of the body.

The fear of this pain explains why heart attacks tend to occur when a vulnerable individual feels the desire for love and is on the verge of making a positive move out of the trap of lovelessness. It is painful to become aware of how empty and unfulfilling one's life has been and may still be. But if that awareness leads to crying, not to more attempts at suppression, the pain is immediately diminished and washed away.

Evoking the pain serves another purpose, namely, arousing the suppressed anger so that it can be directed outward. Because held-in anger in almost all cases is related to the traumas of early childhood, it cannot be expressed against one's parents later in life. If suppressed, it may emerge as rage in reaction to some minor frustration. Unfortunately, such outbursts, as we have seen, do not discharge the anger, which then poses a threat to the heart. Letting it out on one's children, which is a common practice, is "acting out" and provides no real release. Instead, it should be expressed in a proper setting where it can do no harm. Patients in therapy can discharge their held-in anger by beating a bed in the therapist's office or at home. This exercise reduces the tension in the muscles of the back and shoulders, frees the chest, and allows the person to breathe more deeply and fully. Directing the anger outward in this fashion greatly diminishes self-destructive behavior, which, in the final analysis, results from anger being turned against the self.

I have suggested that the wish to die is connected to such major diseases as cancer and heart attack. Why, then, does one person die from cancer while another succumbs to a fatal heart attack? Cancer involves a slow death, and is caused by a gradual erosion of the wish to live. Strangely, the will to live remains fairly strong in cancer patients until the end. While the body is dying, the ego continues to assert its will to live, an assertion that becomes increasingly meaningless as the disease progresses. In effect, the cancer patient does not give up the neurotic struggle until death ends it. But isn't this also true of the heart attack victim? Yes and no. The heart attack victim is more aware of his struggle, and of the desire to give it up. If he can't break free by a deliberate act, he will do something destructive to release himself from his trap, just like the two top executives Friedman discussed who lost their positions by failing to file income tax returns. Still, it is better to lose a position than one's life. In some cases, the heart attack itself is a way of getting out from under intolerable pressures. But it cannot be claimed that the person gave himself an attack; he may have invited it, but if so, he did it unwillingly.

The heart attack victim is caught in a conflict—he wants out, but he is afraid to get out. To get out, he has to open up, which evokes the pain of heartbreak and the fear of abandonment. His death, if it happens through an attack, is not a result of emotional resignation but of fear. Symbolically, the heart attack is like the panic reaction that occurs when an impulse to break out, reach out, and open up becomes strong enough to challenge the seeming security of the status quo. Neither that impulse nor the panic is conscious. If they were, the problem would be transferred to the conscious level, where it could be dealt with. Death from a heart attack also denotes a loss of hope, for the heart is as much the organ of hope as the organ of love. The loss of hope, a sequel to panic, is an overwhelming, acute feeling that is very different from the emotional resignation of the cancer patient, whose hope is slowly eroded by the wish to die.[3]

When these issues can be brought out and discussed in the therapeutic situation, the fear becomes manageable. And since this fear is coupled with loneliness, it is greatly diminished when another person is available with a sympathetic ear. For many patients, the relation to the therapist is a life-supporting connection. Facing one's conflicts is always a painful and frightening experience, but it is also very rewarding, for it holds the potential of a life that is not corrupted by a wish to die.

The following case is interesting because the patient had all the symptoms of a heart attack, without actually having one. I believe that Morris avoided an infarction by remaining in touch with his feelings. The incident occurred when positive feelings of love were trying to break through his armored chest. A clinical pathologist about fifty-five years old, Morris had been in bioenergetic therapy for a number of years. His struggle to open his heart was a main focus of the therapy. He had been married for the third time about ten years earlier, and the relationship during most of that time was tempestuous. Periods of good feeling and warmth between him and his wife, Barbara, would be followed by distancing, coldness, hurt feelings, and angry outbursts. It was a complicated relationship that nevertheless improved slowly as each worked on his personal issues. Morris, for his part, was working hard to be a more autonomous person and not to be dependent on a woman, to be more identified with and secure in his sexuality, and to be a more loving person. The problems he had with Barbara paralleled those he had experienced with his mother. He adopted a helper role and was always "there" for her; and he became furious when, in turn, she was not there for him.

The incident, as Morris recounted it, enables us to understand the feelings and conflicts involved in the attempt to break through the tensions that imprison feelings of the heart. It began with Morris awakening from a dream "with a terrible feeling in my throat and esophagus." In the dream he saw a man he knew whose chest muscles had been ripped open by long cuts. He relates, "I was overcome with grief at this awful sight. I was sure he was going to die, yet I felt wonderful feelings for him. But I arose with that pain in my throat."

The interpretation of the dream is easy. The man in the dream was Morris himself, whose chest and throat were opening, producing some wonderful feelings but also pain and the fear of dying. Once he was wide awake, the pain felt like indigestion, and it got worse as he tried to sit up. He became frightened and wondered if he might be having a heart attack. He broke out into a clammy sweat and thought that he might be dying. At this point, he woke Barbara, saying, "I may be very ill." She decided to call the ambulance, to which Morris agreed, feeling sick, clammy, and on the point of passing out. However, he now had no pain in his throat or chest. The idea that he might be dying persisted, and Morris prepared himself to accept that possibility.

One member of the emergency medical team was the husband of a woman named Jenny who had once been Morris's assistant. Morris asked the man about Jenny and their new baby and learned that they were well. Morris reported, "As I thought about Jenny, I felt my heart and a surge of love for her. I said, 'Tell her I love her.' It felt very important to me."

When Morris got to the hospital, the emergency-room staff immediately hooked him to a monitor, took an EKG, and inserted a tube into his hand. He felt reassured by their prompt actions and impressed by their efficiency. The EKG showed that the heart was normal. However, he was sent to intensive care, where he spent the night hooked to a monitor. The next day, feeling better and realizing that his heart was okay, he and his wife discussed their emotional situation and his "real" heart problem.

He reported the following: In the ambulance, on the way to the hospital, it meant a lot to me to say, "Tell Jenny I love her." I felt my heart; I do love her. In the emergency room, as I looked around, I thought, Whom can I love here? What had been going on is that my wife had not allowed me to love her for the past four weeks. She had been furious with me, jealous because she thought I was taken with another woman. I stood back, keeping my distance and not feeling sexual. As the days went by, I felt something was dying in me. As my wife and I talked in the hospital, I felt I might die for her. What the feeling meant was I would have died for my mother to make her happy or to bring her back to me. I remembered that as a child I was preoccupied with the idea of sacrificing some of my life so that my parents would live hundreds of years. It represented a fear of losing them, for underneath I sensed the feeling that I'd die without them. During the trouble with my wife, I recall crying one night in bed with the same thought—"I'll die without you"—and feeling an ache in my throat. I desperately wanted to call out for someone—for Mother—and I had the terrible knowledge that she would not come, would not hear, that my voice and feelings would be unwelcome. It was a terrible feeling of aloneness, pain, desperation—abandonment, although the word doesn't seem to do justice to the terrible quality of the feeling that I could die. One night during this time, I fell asleep and had two terrible sensations that seemed to go on all night. One was that my throat and esophagus were going to collapse and I'd die; the other was a feeling that if I didn't disguise and hide myself, I'd be killed. I understand that now as having to hide my feelings and needs or be killed. I closed up somehow. That's how I felt when I sensed the rage in my wife and her craziness in accusing me at being involved with another woman. She was in a panic, and it panicked me, which made me realize my mother had been in somewhat the same state. I realized how desperate I was to help her, to help my mother, but I also sensed that I was *helpless*. Being helpless freed me somehow to cry for myself and feel my aloneness. I now felt and admitted how unhappy I had been most of my life, something I had been ashamed to recall, as if I had no right to be unhappy. It was an unhappiness I could never seem to do anything about—because it was my mother's unhappiness. Somehow I had taken it into me and felt it was mine.

A child's identification with his mother's feelings stems from the symbiotic fusion between them. It is not a psychological phenomenon. During the nine months that the child is developing in the womb, his body is in such intimate contact with his mother's that he senses and responds to every wave of feeling that passes through the mother. Even at birth, the infant's body is so attuned to his mother that he vibrates in harmony with her. If a mother is sad and unhappy, her child will feel sad and unhappy. If she is excited and alive, her child will feel the same way. Her feelings determine the mood in the home. If she is unhappy, her unhappiness will cast a pall over the spirits of children and adults alike who live in the house. An adult can leave the house and find some pleasurable excitement elsewhere, but a young child is trapped. He cannot feel good unless his mother feels good, so he must do whatever is in his power to lift his mother's spirits. Inevitably he will fail and become an unhappy, heavy-hearted child. His mother's unhappiness has now become his own. This kind of unhappiness is not the kind a child can discharge by crying. How can he burden his poor, unhappy mother with his sadness when she has so much of her own? Intuitively, the child knows that his mother cannot respond to his needs.

Morris recognized this dilemma. He said, "I realize that I can do something about my unhappiness now—I can cry. This realization is connected to my throat. I've closed off my throat to suppress my crying, which has left me trapped."

Morris's role of helping women was an extension of his role as a boy. It may have also determined his choice of profession. Being there for mother enables a child to overcome the terrible feeling of aloneness and abandonment that threatens his life. Denying himself and assuming responsibility for another becomes a way of survival.

We can see from the above that it is not difficult for a child to become trapped in his relationship to his mother so that separation is not easy to achieve. As an adult, he can become trapped in an unfulfilling relationship by the feeling that it is his role to make his partner happy so that he himself can be fulfilled. But this explanation is only half the story. The cage that imprisons the heart does not fully swing shut until the close of the Oedipal period. A boy who is there for his mother is usually involved in a situation that has sexual undertones and overtones. Morris was aware that his mother had been seductive with him and that her behavior was responsible for what he called his sexual "craziness." He said:

> My mother played with me, teasing, tempting, taunting, holding herself out and then not being available. I could sense that she almost drove me crazy with her seductive behavior. I realize now that a lot of my sexual excitement is tied up with preoccupations, titillations, games, and not in the act of sex itself.

The effect on Morris, as on any child caught in a similar situation, was to create a sense of guilt about his sexuality. One may wonder why he felt guilty in this situation instead of his mother, since he was the injured party. But few parents allow themselves to feel guilty about their seductive behavior with their children. They do not see their behavior as morally wrong or damaging to the child. In their eyes, it is a harmless excitement that they can control so that it doesn't lead to incest. Unfortunately, the child cannot control his excitement. He becomes overstimulated, which is all the more difficult since he has no avenue to release the charge as an adult does. Part of him desperately wants sexual contact with the parent, and part of him is frightened at the prospect and knows it is wrong. Since it is wrong, someone must take the blame. A parent has no trouble making the child feel responsible for his sexual involvement with the parent. By projecting the guilt on the child, the parent denies his culpability. The child has no choice but to accept the guilt, which destroys his innocence and closes the door on his childhood.

We have already seen the consequences of such experiences. In adulthood, sex becomes dissociated from love. The individual may find sexual fulfillment with a casual partner, but it is difficult for him to become highly excited by someone he truly loves. As he learned only too well as a child, such intense feelings toward a love object are taboo.

But dissociating sex from love places the heart in danger because it cannot fulfill its deepest longings. The solution is to become a loving person whose heart is open to a full range of feelings. To accomplish that, it is necessary to live by principles that maintain the integrity of the personality. We shall examine some of these principles in the next chapter.

CHAPTER 10

The Healthy Heart—The Loving Person

The Heart has its reasons which reason will never know.
Pascal

There is a growing realization today that heart disease is related to one's attitudes and patterns of behavior. Consequently, health-conscious people are trying not only to diminish the stresses of modern living but to strengthen the body to withstand these stresses. For many, physical fitness is the name of the game. They watch their diet, exercise regularly, stop smoking, have regular medical checkups, and sometimes engage in meditation or other relaxation techniques. While all these practices are to be recommended, they fail to address the key issue leading to heart disease that we have examined in this book, namely, the lack of love. It is my thesis that a person whose heart is open to love will not develop coronary artery disease. Such a person will not be rigid, will breathe fully, and will not be drawn to achieve or perform like a Type A personality. If this assessment is valid, those of us concerned about the health of our hearts should focus our interest on how we can open them up to love.

The problem most of us face is that the defenses we erected to protect the heart have become its prison and are now unconscious. Many individuals are not even aware of the tension in their chest or of their inability to open their heart. Most people believe that they would be fully capable of loving if only they were loved. They confuse the longing for love with loving itself. They sense love in their hearts but can't get to it, cut off as they are from their hearts by the barriers they erected to save it.

It is not enough to make a decision to be more loving. We can no more force ourselves to feel love than we can make ourselves happy by an effort of will. Feelings by their very nature arise from deep within the organism, and though we can dull or suppress them, we are impotent to create them. While it is true that one can evoke a feeling through fantasy or by acting the feeling, it is not the genuine article unless the action touches a suppressed reservoir of emotion. Occasionally one can break through the barriers that hold back the feeling of love so that it reaches the surface, but such breakthrough experiences, important as they are, do not change the personality if the barriers are not understood and removed. Many people, for example, have experienced the overwhelming joy of falling in love. In many cases, though, the love has a childish or romantic quality and collapses in the face of adult reality, leaving the person as closed to love as he was when he began.

In order to open the heart so that it gives meaning to the person and life to the body, we need to determine why and how it got closed off and what forces and fears keep it locked up. Without this knowledge and understanding, therapists cannot dismantle the armor or remove the barricades either for ourselves or our patients. The first step is to investigate and analyze the person's past, especially the experiences of childhood. At the same time, we must foster an understanding of the physical processes that armor the individual. We need to see the body not in a mechanical way but as the living expression of an individual's history. As we have seen, every chronic tension in the body is a sign of some early conflict that has left the person with an unresolved fear. These fears need to be worked through and eliminated if he is to keep his heart open to life. To do this, muscular tensions must be released and suppressed feelings allowed to reach consciousness. Both processes, the analytic and the physical, proceed side by side in therapy, as they do in life.

The following vignette from a therapy session shows these interconnections. While the patient, a woman in her thirties whom I will call Barbara, was lying on the bed, I suggested that she reach out with her arms and say what she wanted. She said, "I want to feel love in my heart." She had in mind, she told me later, her husband and her sisters. Her statement of desire brought up a feeling of sadness, but she could not cry. Her tight, grim jaw and her tense body made it very difficult for her to melt with tears. As we discussed her inability to cry, she added, "I have the same problem when I'm in bed with my husband and begin to soften with sexual desire. I stiffen, cut off the feeling, and become hostile." She explained, "If I allow my feelings to show, I feel people will enjoy them and will get some perverse pleasure from my helplessness." Then she added, "If you lose control, you are upstaged." I added to myself, "And humiliated."

Barbara had complained earlier about a lack of privacy in her childhood. She felt strongly that her mother was always watching her and that her father was very conscious of her sexuality. As an adult, Barbara still acted as if any show of feeling would expose her to humiliation. Of course, she knew that wasn't the case, but her conscious mind could not override the feeling of fear, which was structured in the chronic tensions of her body.

Feeling, as we pointed out earlier, is the perception of what goes on in the body. In Barbara's case, the suppression of feeling signaled a fear of exposure and humiliation. If she cried, it was inevitable that she would feel humiliated, since humiliation was the feeling she was seeking to suppress. But if she never cried, she would always fear exposure and humiliation. Was the position a trap? Not if Barbara could find the courage to test her adult reality. The feeling of humiliation that she might experience as she gave way to crying would be momentary. It would change quickly to a feeling of relief with the realization that those close to her would respond to her crying with sympathy and understanding.

Since Barbara wanted that relief, it was not too difficult to help her yield. I asked her to reach again and this time to ask for my help. Despite her desperate need, this gesture was hard for her to do with feeling. As she said the words "Please help me," I applied some pressure to the sides of her jaw, which caused them to relax. In less than a minute, Barbara began to sob. When she finished crying, she remarked how good it felt to be able to let go. She knew that she could not have done it without my intervention.

In that she is not alone. Many people are paralyzed by the conflicting pull of "I want to" and "I won't" and need the intervention of a therapist to shift the balance from the suppression of feeling to its expression.

Small children are the exception. When a baby is frightened, hurt, or frustrated, his jaw begins to quiver, which leads immediately into deep sobbing. This is both a cry of distress and the convulsive discharge of tension.

As the baby grows older, he learns other ways to discharge tension. One is to become angry when he is injured or insulted. For example, a child frightened by an unexpected movement may strike out at the person who startled him. The expression of anger manifested in a physical attack discharges the tension. The child also learns to release by getting away from a stressful situation. As he gets older, he may also turn to laughter.

None of these choices is available to infants, for whom crying is the only way to release tension. Crying is also the only way for adults to relieve the tension that results from the loss of love. The process of mourning is ineffective to discharge the pain of loss unless it includes sobbing deeply. One can also get angry at the death of a loved one, as primitive people sometimes

do, but their anger is always accompanied by wailing, screaming, and crying. One of my patients told me that following the
death of his wife some years ago, he cried every night for a
week. The pain of the loss was so great he did not believe he
would survive it. But crying let him sleep, which gave him the
energy to go on.

Whereas anger releases the tension along the back of the
body, crying releases the tension along the front. Each sob is
like a pulse that arises deep in the abdomen (belly crying) and
passes upward through the chest and throat, to be released as
sound. To emit the sound, one has to breathe out; crying is
impossible if one holds one's breath. Blocking the sound by
tension in the throat and jaw will also inhibit crying. But if
these impediments are overcome, the chest feels lighter and
breathing is easier after a good cry.

Laughter is very similar to crying in its tension-releasing
ability. As we have seen, Norman Cousins encourages the use of
laughter as an antidote to panic and an aid to healing. Its
positive values can hardly be denied; it lifts one's spirits. Physi-
ologically, laughter and crying are not very different; both are
convulsive reactions in which the voice is used and breathing
mobilized. The release of tension results from the convulsive
movements of the body, but where laughter ends in an upward
turn of the face, crying turns the face downward. A good belly
laugh and a good belly cry are not the same psychologically. To
laugh when one feels sad does nothing to discharge the sadness,
though it may temporarily release us. Only crying deeply
discharges the sadness.

Many patients laugh as a way of blocking or denying their
sadness. Sometimes a patient will start laughing spontaneously
as he breathes deeply while bent back over the stool, but
laughter is inappropriate, since there is nothing funny or hu-
morous in the situation. But if one encourages the person to
keep the laughter going, one may find that it turns suddenly
into crying. It can happen the other way, too. I recall an

incident when this occurred. My wife was working on the tension in my shoulders while I was seated on the floor. Standing behind me, she pressed her fists into the tight muscles between my neck and shoulders. It was so painful that I began to cry. Then, suddenly, the pain disappeared, and I was laughing. When the muscles let go, the tension went out of them, and so did the pain. I was laughing with relief and good feeling.

Some people find it very hard to cry and even pride themselves on their ability to "take it" without breaking down. There are times and places where such an attitude is sign of bravery. Not to break down before an enemy is commendable, but to carry this attitude into ordinary life is foolish and dangerous. One might well ask whether the person is trying to prove that he is made of stone. But in these cases, as in so many others, the real reasons lie under the surface, in the unconscious. Not crying was the way they survived as children. By not crying, the child can deny a punishing and hostile parent the satisfaction of knowing he made the child submit. By turning to stone, the child can make a parent feel powerless. No one is powerful enough to bend a stone to his will. In addition, many men feel ashamed of crying. If they do cry, they cover their face with their hands. On a conscious level, they feel it is unmanly to cry. But the difficulty they feel in crying has its origins in their unconscious rigidity, which blocks deep breathing and represents suppressed conflicts.

I mentioned earlier my own difficulty in crying. I was aware for many years that my chest was tight and that it harbored panic. I knew that I had a fear of abandonment. The therapy I had and the exercises I did greatly diminished the panic and fear, but I knew that I was still a candidate for a heart attack. In fact, I dreamed that I would have a heart attack and die. Although no time was given for the attack, the dream did not suggest that it would take place in the distant future. Yet I felt no fear at the prospect. I simply said, "It's all right so long as I die with dignity." The following night I dreamed that I was the trusted adviser to an infant king. He believed that I had betrayed him and ordered my execution. I was led to the place of execution where my head would be cut off. I saw the executioner standing with his ax beside the block, but I felt no fear, for I was sure that the king would realize his error and free me at the last minute. The seconds ticked away, the time of execution approached, and no reprieve came. At the last moment, I looked down and saw that the chain binding my leg was tinsel and that I could just walk away. At that I awoke. The vividness of the dream indicated that it was important.

As I thought about the dream, its meaning became clear to me. The infant king was my heart; the trusted adviser was my head. My head had betrayed my heart by assuming power and dictating behavior on the ground that the king, my heart, was infantile. The dream depicted the typical conflict between the adult ego and the heart. If I would save my heart, I had to lose my head—that was one message of the dream. The other was that there was no real threat to my life if I saw the reality of my situation. I was free. I simply had to acknowledge the hegemony of my heart. I had created the conflict and therefore could resolve it by realizing that the role of the adviser is not to make decisions. That is the king's prerogative. The role of the adviser is to keep the king informed and help him implement his decisions. I would describe the head-heart relationship as follows: The heart will tell you what to do, and the head will tell you the best way to do it.

My approach to the problem discussed in this book—namely, the inability to open the heart to love—is both psychological and physical. On the psychological level, it is necessary for the person to understand the nature of the problem and gain as much insight into its cause as he can. This involves a careful analysis to help him get in touch with the experiences of his childhood. But I don't believe that analysis alone is fully effective. The problem is structured in the body in the form of chronic muscular tensions, as I have pointed out many times in this book. I have described the armoring in the front of the chest that blocks the longing and the carapace on the back that immobilizes the expression of anger. These tensions must be released to a significant degree if healthy functioning is to be established. The first step in a treatment program is to see these tensions.

Figure 14A is a drawing taken from a photograph of a depressed forty-three-year-old male patient who had suffered a myocardial infarction two years earlier. The curvature of the back is the most evident feature in the drawing. Some animals manifest this kind of hump when they are so angry that the hair stands erect on their backs. Like them, this man had his back up. About four weeks before the attack he had been called out on the carpet by his superior, which he described as a very humiliating experience. Though angry and furious, he did not express his feelings. During the ensuing Christmas holidays, he felt tired and restless at the same time. He also experienced some difficulty in breathing. He looked so haggard that he was advised to take a vacation. Over the New Year holidays, he went to California to vacation at his sister's home, and while there, his niece's fiancé, a young man about twenty-one or twenty-two years old, suggested a game of racquetball. The patient couldn't resist the challenge. He lost the first game 21–12 and lost the second one, as well. In the third game he exerted himself strongly but lost again. After the third trouncing, he walked around for fifteen or twenty minutes. When he sat down, he experienced chest pain. Fortunately, the hospital was only five minutes away.

While the curvature of the back is striking, we should not overlook the inflated, armored chest, which denotes heartbreak and panic. Because of his curved back, the inflation of his chest might not be visible if the patient were dressed. Undressed, it is clearly manifest in the exaggerated diameter of the thorax. This patient had never married and had never had a lasting or

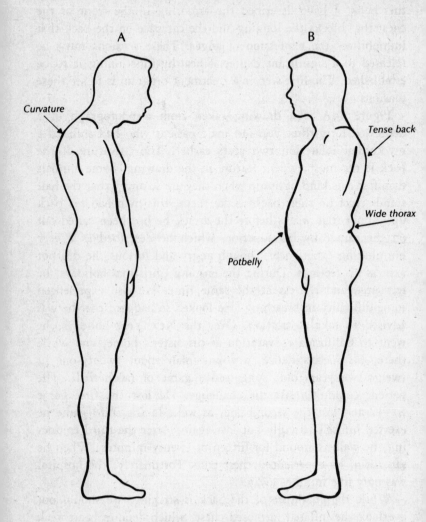

Curvature

Tense back

Wide thorax

Potbelly

A

B

Figure 14. Tension patterns in armored individuals

fulfilling relationship with a woman. In discussing his child-hood, he showed no awareness that he had suffered a loss of love. He recalled very little of his childhood, but he did not believe that there had been anything unusual in his upbringing. Talking about his heart attack evoked no feeling of sadness or any sense that something terrible had happened to him. He recognized that he was angry, but he felt that he was angry with himself for being a failure. By denying any sadness at the lack or loss of love, he had no desire to cry. He could not remember the last time he had cried. Even at the death of his mother some years ago, tears had come to his eyes, but he had never broken down and sobbed.

Figure 14B is the drawing of a fairly common body structure among middle-aged men. It shows the raised, tense back, the exaggerated front-to-back diameter of the thorax, and the fairly typical paunch. A person with this type of body may be a heavy eater and have a high blood cholesterol level. However, these physical features, in my opinion, are secondary to the emotional factors and to the respiratory problems manifested in the en-larged thorax. One other aspect of these drawings merits atten-tion: the collapse of the backside. In both drawings, the buttocks are relatively flattened out, a position suggestive of a dog with its tail between its legs. I regard this bodily attitude as signify-ing a loss of cockiness, another factor in the predisposition to heart disease. Since the person *is* his body, his body has to change if there is to be a dependable change in personality. A description of some of the exercises used to achieve such a change follows.

The basic technique I used to help a person unblock his crying is to mobilize his breathing and his voice. There are several ways this can be done, but in treating people who have hardened themselves, it is helpful to use a bioenergetic stool. The stool, which is shown in figure 15, measures twenty-four inches high. A rolled-up blanket with a paper core is strapped to the top. The person lies back on the stool, his arms stretched above his head toward a chair. The blanket makes contact opposite the nipple line. This position is adapted from the tension-relieving stretch people so often take when they've been sitting too long. To get a few good breaths, they lift their torsos and stretch their arms up over the back of the chair. Since most people suffer from significant tension in the muscles of the back, this position on the stool is uncomfortable. However, if the person relaxes as much as possible, the stool helps him to breathe by stretching the tight muscles surrounding the thorax. It is difficult to hold one's breath while lying over the stool, and individuals who are rigid will sense both their rigidity and their inability to breathe deeply. (A more complete description of how the stool can be used will be found in the bioenergetic manual of exercises.[1])

As we have seen, people who hold in their feelings hold in their breath. Lying over the stool promotes breathing out and so favors "letting go." If one breathes out, with a deep abdominal expiration, the suppressed sadness cannot be held and will erupt spontaneously. In most cases, people cannot breathe that deeply, but such breathing can be furthered by the use of the voice. Sustaining a moderate sound while lying over the stool will deepen the expiration if one makes the effort. The inability to sustain a sound for more than a few seconds is a sign of respiratory difficulty, even though one may not feel this difficulty in normal life. Usually, respiratory distress is associated with difficulty in breathing in, whereas here the problem is the inability to breathe out deeply. Most people will stop the sound as it reaches the breaking point, that is, the point where a continued expiration would result in a discontinuous sound like "uh, uh, uh," which could easily break into sobbing. In many cases, bronchial tension causes the person to cough. If tension in the throat is severe, he will begin to choke. In some cases, the feeling of sadness is swallowed back as it wells up. Whatever form the resistance takes, I encourage the person to let go as much as possible and to deliberately make crying sounds. Even

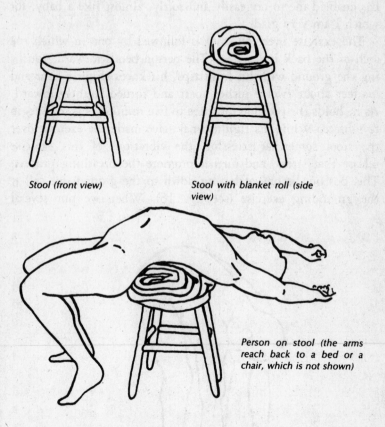

Stool (front view)

Stool with blanket roll (side view)

Person on stool (the arms reach back to a bed or a chair, which is not shown)

Figure 15. The bioenergetic stool and the breathing exercise

so, it still is not easy for many people, especially men, to break down and cry. It wasn't easy for me, either. I was frightened of the pain in my heart, but I realized how important it was for me to be able to cry. Working with my breathing over the years has enabled me to cry easily and softly, almost like a baby, for which I am very glad.

The exercise over the stool is followed by one in which the arch of the back is reversed. The person bends forward, touching the ground with his fingertips, his knees slightly bent and his feet about twelve inches apart and turned slightly inward. As he holds the position for three to five minutes, his legs begin to vibrate. While his rigidity may have made the exercise over the stool somewhat stressful, the vibrations of this exercise release that stress, and further promote the breathing process. This position is one of letting down to the ground; we call it the grounding exercise (see fig. 16). When we put several

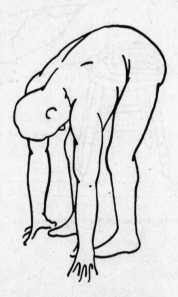

Figure 16. The grounding exercise

cardiac patients at a workshop through these exercises, all of them reported feeling easier and better afterward.

It isn't necessary to use a bioenergetic stool to deepen one's breathing. One can lie on the floor over a rolled-up blanket placed under the upper back. While this position is not as effective as lying over the stool, one can evoke crying by using the voice as described above. Even using the voice while sitting in a chair can help a person to cry. Recalling some sadness or loss in one's life is helpful. Many people say that they can cry watching a sad show on television or listening to music, but in most cases they are talking about tears rather than sobs. While tears are important, both as an expression of sadness and as cleansing agent for the eyes, they do not serve to release the tension resulting from a loss of love. For that purpose we need to cry throatily and uncontrollably.

In bioenergetic therapy we use another exercise to help people express the feeling of protest common to everyone who has suffered the loss of a loved one. Many primitives scream their protest when a loved one dies, but we sophisticated and civilized people accept death and loss philosophically, even though this rational attitude denies the body's feelings and deadens our emotional life. The exercise consists of having the patient lie on a bed on his back and kick the bed rhythmically with outstretched legs. If the bed has a four- or five-inch foam mattress, he can kick as hard as he wants without hurting himself or damaging the bed. As he kicks, the patient shouts in a loud and sustained voice, "Why?" I ask patients to shout three "whys," sustaining each one until the breath is gone while kicking continues, at which point he draws another breath. As the exercise moves from the first "why" to the third, the kicking is speeded up and the voice is raised. Many women will end the third "why" in a scream. Crying and screaming are part of a true mourning process. This exercise discharges the tension in the chest, throat, and legs and significantly deepens the breathing so that one is very conscious of its spontaneity. Like deep crying, screaming or shouting a strong protest lifts the weight of sadness and pain off the heart.

The important thing about these exercises is that their effect on respiration is not limited to the period of the exercise. Because they help the person overcome his fear of surrendering to his feelings, they can produce far-reaching and long-lasting changes in behavior and personality. Instead of holding feelings in, the patient learns to let go, to be looser, softer, and freer. This happens more readily when the person is in a form of therapy that allows him to probe his memory for an understanding of the forces that have made him uptight. But it should be emphasized that therapy is not an absolute requirement for growth and maturation. Life provides many occasions for us to express our feelings openly and directly, and each time we do so, we learn to be a more open and loving person. But exercises such as these help greatly in the process of opening our hearts and expressing our feelings.

Any discussion of our feelings is not complete if it omits the problem of anger. Most people are not generally conscious of held-in anger, despite the fact that they may feel irritable or explode in a rage from time to time. Nor are they aware of the enormous tension in the upper back that accompanies suppressed anger. A person's back may be up, but generally he doesn't feel it. As we have seen, this suppressed anger stems from early childhood experiences of deprivation, denial, and the need to submit to parental authority. In many cases, these early experiences include physical abuse by a parent in the name of punishment. The anger in response to such abuse is so intense that it verges on murderous rage, which most people are reluctant to give in to out of fear that they might lose control and seriously hurt someone. But when such feelings are held in, the person turns them against himself and becomes self-destructive. Such held-in anger also makes it very difficult for a person to ask for what he wants or to say no to an unreasonable demand. He is afraid that should he meet with resistance, he would explode in rage.

And so he carries this anger in the form of chronic muscular tension, like a monkey on his back. If he is to deal easily and rationally with stressful situations, the anger must be vented. The logical way is for him to strike a bed with all his fury, using whatever words seem appropriate. While this exercise provides a cathartic release, its prime purpose is to free up the shoulders and arms so that they can reach out softly for love. Anger that has been held in for years cannot be discharged with one exercise. As long as the "monkey" sits on his back, the person will be an angry individual. Two things are necessary to accomplish a full release: One, the person must feel and identify with his anger; and, two, he must continue the hitting as a regular exercise at home until he is free from tension in his back and shoulders. (See *The Way to Vibrant Health* for directions on how to do this exercise.)

The routine I follow every morning after washing up and before breakfast is to lie over the stool for several minutes to allow my body to stretch and my breathing to deepen. I lie in different positions, working my way down from my upper to my lower back. These positions are uncomfortable despite all the years that I have worked with the stool. They cannot be comfortable so long as there is any tension in the muscles of the back or in the shoulder girdle. For many people, though, they are downright painful because of the tension in the back muscles. Some people may fear their back may break, which won't happen, but no one should stay in a painful position if it is too frightening. The pain, though, is not a negative sign, as it represents the conflict between the wish to let go and the fear of doing so. The pain can always be decreased by moaning or groaning, which releases some of the tension by deepening the breathing.

After I work with the stool, I do the grounding exercise described above. After my legs start to vibrate, my whole body feels more charged and alive. At this point, I perform some hitting or other exercises involving my arms and shoulders. And from time to time I let myself cry when I realize how rigid I have been and how much my life has been a struggle. As long as I can cry, I know my body is soft and my heart is open. This routine has helped me reach the point where I can discharge my pent-up anger and give up being an angry man.

The surprising result is that my anger is readily available to me. I can feel it surge when I believe that someone has taken advantage of me. I can express it with my eyes so that people can see that I am angry without my having to attack them. Having access to my anger has made me feel more of a person, and because I am more often treated that way, I have less need to be angry. I am also less afraid since I am less vulnerable and less defensive since I am more open in my mind and in my heart.

If we talk about a healthy heart, we must realize that it exists only in a healthy person. If we are to heal a broken heart, the role that love plays in life must be made clear. In this an analogy may be helpful. I have described the heart as the hub of a wheel in which the spokes represent the impulses of love from the heart. These impulses, like spokes, support the rim or boundary of the individual. Just as a wheel can't operate without a rim, a person can't function without a boundary demarcating the self.

When I work with a person to help him open his heart, I do not suggest that he surrender all his defenses. To do so would reduce him to the level of an infant, who may be all heart but who is also dependent and helpless. This is why it is so important to help a person feel and identify with his anger. If he has ways to fight back, he does not need to lock himself in a fortress as way of protection. Nor does he need to remain in a painful situation.

In chapter 3 I discussed the stages of growth and described how the personality becomes split into two centers, the heart and the ego. We will review those stages (see figs. 9 and 10.) in terms of the quality of love each represent.

Love = desire for closeness and contact.

a. Infantile love .... needs warmth, nurturing, support, and protection;
in return, offers connection to future beyond self; renewal and rebirth

b. Child love .... needs support, protection, and approval;
in return, shares joy of play

c. Boy or girl love ..... needs support, approval, and guidance;
in return, shares excitement of adventure and offers deep friendships

d. Youthful love .... needs guidance and freedom;
in return, offers excitement and thrill of romance and sex

e. Adult love .... needs a mate to share life;
in return, gives affection, respect, and support

The above is a fair representation of how love evolves as the person develops and matures. When that development is hampered by heartbreaking events in childhood, the impulse to love is restricted and comes through hesitantly, tentatively, and halfheartedly. The degree of restriction varies according to the timing and severity of those early experiences. As a result, the impulse to love carries with it unfulfilled needs from earlier stages. The words "I love you" could mean (a) "I need your nurturing;" (b) "I need your support;" (c) "I need your approval;" (d) "I need your sexual response to me;" or (e) "I want to share my life with you." For some people, love has a strong infantile element; for others, it contains a large romantic element. When these early elements are strong, the mature element is diminished. Thus, when a patient talks of feelings of love for a spouse or a partner, I want to know from what layer of personality he or she is speaking. I evaluate the statement of love in terms of the individual's degree of maturity.

In treating a person for any emotional problem, it is not enough to focus only on the heart. If we concentrate on the whole person, understanding that love is central to his problem, we can help him open his heart and find the fulfillment in love that he seeks. One of my patients, a man in his early forties whom I will call Michael, had a number of disappointing and frustrating experiences with women despite the fact that his main aim in life was to find love. Michael was a strong, vital, and good-looking man to whom many women were attracted. He responded to them warmly, since he felt that life without the love of a woman was empty. Still, his marriage had failed, and three other extended relationships had collapsed. He was looking for an ideal woman, one who would fulfill all his unfulfilled needs. But every time he possessed a woman's love, he saw only how she failed to live up to his ideal. On the other hand, if a woman refused to give him her full commitment, he became hung up on her and went through some very painful feelings. Mightn't she, after all, have been the ideal one? A woman's unavailability evoked the same taboo feelings he felt for his mother.

This analysis, though valid, was not the factor that helped Michael change. He knew about his involvement with his mother. What he didn't know was how this involvement had fixated him at the level of a boy. I pointed out to Michael that his issue was to become a man, not to find love. With time, he came to understand how he had betrayed himself in his relationships with women, just as he had been betrayed by his mother into being her "little man." This awareness brought up anger at his mother and at all women and the strong feeling that he didn't need anything from them. Not needing allowed him to love as a man—wholeheartedly.

To reach this point takes considerable analysis. After the heartbreaks of childhood, the personality develops with many twists and turns. Rarely are adults direct and open; more often they are indirect and defensive, submissive and resentful. This has to be worked through. One of the exercises I use is aimed at helping a person say "no." Lying on a bed with his legs extended, he is instructed to kick as hard as he can. At the same time, I encourage him to say "no," as loud and as long as possible. Sustaining the word "no" in this way has a powerful effect on the breathing and also helps to release feeling. If a person is not blocked or inhibited in his self-assertion, the "no" comes out loud and clear. But this is not always the case. Most people find it difficult to express themselves forcefully without first being provoked. They were not allowed to assert themselves as children and have trouble doing so as adults. This exercise provides a way to confront the problem and, by practicing, learn to overcome it. One can also say "no" standing up, either to a therapist or to a group, as a form of assertiveness training.

The ability to say "no" is the mark of a secure individual. The insecure individual acts out his "no" by not doing what he has been asked to do and then excusing himself by claiming that he forgot. His forgetfulness may be real, but it is a symptom of hostility. The same applies to the person who says "yes" submissively. Though he may try to hide his resentment, it will show in many small ways that the other person will sense. On the other hand, saying "no" openly and directly indicates trust in the other person. Without the belief that the other will understand and accept one's feelings, it is impossible to share the self.

Generally, an honest "no" is more easily accepted. The other person may not be happy with the refusal, but he or she appreciates the respect and trust such a "no" expresses. An honest "yes" or "I love you" coming from the same person has all the more impact. Too often the words "I love you" are used to avoid a conflict or to cover up hostility. For many people it is not love but a fear of abandonment that keeps them in a relationship. In such a context, the statement "I love you" does not mean what it says.

What we have said here about saying "no" openly and directly applies to any relationship that involves trust. The man who can't say "no" to his boss is neither trusted nor respected because his submissiveness is based on fear. Moreover, the denial of the self inherent in a submissive attitude undermines a person's ability to be creative or innovative. "Yes" men may be skilled in carrying out orders, but they are lost if required to think on their feet.

In any relationship, it is not a question of having one's way but of having one's say. We all recognize that a lack of communication is a problem in relationships. But just as we don't speak up and express our true feelings, so we don't hear what others have to say. We hear the words, but too often we take them as a personal attack, not as the affirmation of another person's feelings. By closing our minds, we also close our hearts. In that case, the situation degenerates into a conflict that only the use of power can resolve. The other person may submit to us, or we to him, to maintain the relationship. By behaving this way, however, we are perpetuating the pattern in our childhood home, where mother's or father's "no" was always the final word.

Clearly, an open mind, an open heart, and a willingness to listen are essential to the loving person. So is a personality that integrates the head and the heart with sexuality (see fig. 11, in chap. 11). We saw in chapter 1 that the intimate connection between these segments is disrupted in many people, so that thinking is dissociated from feeling and sexuality from love. This disruption destroys the integrity of the personality, so that how one behaves in business bears no relation to how one treats one's family. Love thy neighbor may be a meaningful doctrine in church on Sunday but irrelevant in the office on Monday. Similarly, when one's life is compartmentalized, an affair with a secretary or colleague in no way contradicts the love one professes for one's wife. But to be a different person in different situations means not to be a whole person in any of them. One may feel loving feelings, but they are limited and imperfect.

What does it mean to be a whole, loving person? Generally in matters of love, the head cannot dictate to the heart. One cannot decide whom to love or even when to fall in love. In many cases, the head would not choose the same love object as the heart, but who listens to his head where love is concerned? Cool reason never prevails in the heat of passion. Does this mean that we will make a mistake if we follow our heart's desire? I don't believe so. It is true that in the height of passion we tend to idealize the person we love, but there is something remarkable in the fact that he or she can excite us to such heights. Unfortunately, when we come down to earth, we may be confronted by a different reality—problems, shortcomings, and all sorts of human frailties. Does that mean that love was blind? Not necessarily.

In chapter 3 we saw that the personality becomes split into two separate centers, the heart and the ego, as a result of the early loss of love. As a defensive gesture, the ego encloses the heart in a protective cage and examines everyone who might reach it with a critical and cynical eye. But all the while, the heart is looking for someone to love, someone to set it free. When it finds that person, it overthrows its captor and escapes its prison. Because the heart's eye is unerring, it always finds the right person, but it does not always remain free. When the nuptial flight is over, when lovers have to face the reality of daily life, the ego assumes command and reestablishes the state of protective custody.

The failure of erotic love to maintain its initial intensity does not diminish its significance in human life. Though the fire ignited between two lovers may not burn so brightly over time, it does not die out. It burns strongly at the core, and flashes of it can still be seen in the eyes of the lovers over a lifetime of being together. Nor should we forget that it explodes in moments of ecstasy when the two come together sexually. No, it is not the nature of erotic love but the split in the human personality that accounts for the failure of love relationships. The notion that love can set us free is an illusion, its roots in the childhood belief that if mother loved us unconditionally, life would be paradise. In fact, the rare child who is the object of his mother's unconditional love does enjoy the human equivalent of heavenly bliss. Most of us yearn for that love but never receive it. Even so, the yearning we felt as children survives in our heart and underlies our belief that love will set us free. That it can do so temporarily is a tribute to love's power. But we can only be free, truly free, when love pervades our whole being— when we have become, in fact, a loving person.

To become a loving person, we need to heal the split between the ego and the heart. This does not mean that the ego must abdicate its position as the arbiter of reality or that the head must surrender its hegemony in the hierarchy of the personality but that the head and the heart must work together to promote the health and happiness of the person. We must recognize that power and love are antithetical pursuits and values. Power creates inequalities; its use demands a suspension of feeling. Love, in contrast, is based on a recognition of equality. Even the relationship of a mother to her child must include the acknowledgment that the child is as much a person as she is. Lacking that, the child will develop a narcissistic character structure and will not be able to see others as equals.

Power often contaminates the intimate relationships of adults, undermining the trust essential for love to flourish. Its most common token is money. Many people use money to control and dominate others by giving it or withholding it to enforce their demands. Many people also believe that money can buy love. Love, though, is never one of money's rewards; instead, money often stands in love's way.

The possession of money or power does not necessarily prevent a person from loving in the full sense of the word. Nor does achieving success or fame. However, if the pursuit of these goals dominates the personality, the ego is split off from the heart, and the person is incapable of loving with his whole being. The drive for power, success, or fame requires channeling an inordinate amount of energy to these ends. But channeling energy rigidifies the body, and the rigid body does not easily melt with love. The vulnerability of the Type A personality to heart disease is directly related to the rigidity associated with the drive to succeed. It is also associated, as we have seen, with hostility, panic, and heartbreak. We can focus on one or the other aspect of this problem, but the consequences to the body are much the same.

It does not follow that if a person is oriented to pleasure, he cannot have money, success, or fame. Pleasure is inherent in the creative process,[2] and a loving person is highly creative simply because his heart is in everything he does. He may gain power, fame, and success, but these values do not dominate him. Nor will he sacrifice his integrity to them.

Certain ego values—respect, dignity, honesty, fairness—harmonize with values of the heart and help promote the integrity of the personality. Respect is essential in any love relationship between mature adults. In the absence of self-respect, the feeling of love has an infantile or childish quality, expressing more the need for support and nurturing than the sharing of good feelings. In the absence of respect for the partner, the relationship degenerates into one of convenience. Only the individual to whom respect is important can be a loving person. This is not to say that such a person will never feel angry toward his mate. We noted in chapter 1 that ambivalent feelings are common enough in love relationships. But ambivalence always results in a loss of respect of one person for the other, which eventually undermines the relationship. Self-respect and respect for the other demands that one confront the situation and express one's anger so that the relationship can be restored to solid ground.

Dignity, the outward expression of self-esteem, is another ego value that keeps love rich. It brings a high degree of charge to the personality, which is attractive. Because the dignified individual holds himself proudly erect, many people confuse dignity with rigidity, but they are not the same. The rigid person holds himself up out of a fear of breaking down. The dignified person has no fear of breaking down—he is neither stiff nor stuck up, and he is able to cry. His behavior merits our respect and promises that we will in turn be treated with respect.

Because it represents a state of inner integrity, honesty is another trait that characterizes the loving person. The person whose head and heart are divided speaks out of both sides of his mouth. Any declarations of love he makes are belied by the distrust and suspicion he radiates. Nor is he honest with himself. Instead, he covers up his negative attitude or justifies it by blaming others. But every lie he tells further splits his personality, since his heart knows the truth. Every lie also frays his connection to other people, since he can't have an open heart and lie at the same time.

Unfortunately, few of us have escaped the traumas of childhood, which forced us to isolate our hearts and armor ourselves against love. Still, we all yearn for love, though we cannot fully open our hearts until we feel secure. We will not find that security in the love of another but only in the love we feel for ourselves. Such self-love is not narcissism, as I pointed out in a previous study.[3] Nor is it selfishness. When the feeling of love, of reaching out, extends through the whole body, we experience it as self-love because it gives us pleasure. When that feeling touches another person, we know the joy of loving another, or what psychologists call "object love." But the two are really one, as Erich Fromm says: "We ourselves are the 'object' of our feelings and attitudes; the attitudes toward others and toward ourselves, far from being contradictory, are basically *conjunctive*." Thus, he notes, "An attitude of love toward themselves will be found in all those who are capable of loving others."[4] But we can only love ourselves if respect, dignity, and honesty are the values we live by.

Connecting head and heart is one half of the task of becoming a loving person. The other half is to connect the heart to the genitals so that sexual activity becomes heartfelt. In reality, there is a blood connection between heart and genitals; otherwise, we couldn't be aroused sexually. But since we do not feel the flow of blood, we are not consciously aware of that connection. Feeling the connection between the two depends instead on the depth of our breathing. If we can't connect love and sex, we restrict our breathing to the upper part of the body and hold our breath in. Letting the breath out fully is a prerequisite of giving in to sexuality. It is when our breathing extends deep into the pelvis and reaches the pelvic floor that we sense the connection between thorax and pelvis. In this case, sexual arousal, when it occurs, is not limited to the genitals but includes lovely warm and melting sensations in the pelvis. When sexual feelings are not restricted to the genitals, they are whole-bodied and therefore wholehearted. Some people believe that sexual excitement naturally diminishes with increasing intimacy, but I believe this applies only to the excitement of foreplay. End pleasure, or the satisfaction of orgasm, increases with intimacy, because one can surrender more fully in the security of love.

My focus on love and sexuality may lead some readers to wonder whether I have not ignored the spiritual aspect of love. What about the love of God? Isn't it God I love if I find joy in His creation? Can the love of God be separated from the love of His creatures?

Throughout this book I have emphasized the importance of an integrated being. To talk of spirituality as something separate from all other human functions is to split the unity of the personality. In my view, spirituality is the opposite side of sexuality; both stem from the heart. By looking upward, we reach to the heavens; by looking down, we contact the earth. But with trees, our reach upward can be no stronger than our contact with the earth. Can we truly be spiritual if we are not sexual? I don't believe so.

If the great mystics and religious teachers are right, God resides in the heart. If we put our hearts fully into any activity, it becomes a spiritual expression, an expression of our spirit. Seen in this light, sexuality, when it is a direct expression of love, is God-given and godlike. By the same token, union with God or a merger with cosmic consciousness can have a sexual feeling. When a woman enters a Catholic order, consecrating her life to religious devotion, she becomes the bride of Christ. I like to think that when our hearts are fully open, we are spiritual in our sexuality and sexual in our spirituality.

I started this book with a discussion of the nature of love, which I said is at the heart of life. As we grow and develop, our love changes, embracing more of the world and maturing as we assume more responsibility for those we love. A loving person loves life, and all that is alive and everything that sustains life. It is this love that furthers the ongoing process of life: human, animal, and plant. Responsibility doesn't mean being burdened or being obligated. It means responding with love, but never as a duty. Duty and love are incompatible, since love is the response of a free man whose duty, if anything, is to be a loving person.

CHAPTER 1
1. Kitzup Sh'lh, quoted in Edith B. Schnapper, *The Inward Odyssey* (London: George Allen and Unwin Ltd., 1965), 141.
2. Kaivalya Upanishad, quoted in Schnapper, op. cit., 130.
3. George A. Maloney, *Prayer of the Heart* (Notre Dame, Ind.: Ave Maria Press, 1983), 25.
4. Brother David Steindl-Rast, *Gratefulness: The Heart of Prayer* (New York: Paulist Press, 1984), 31.
5. Chandaya Upanishad, 8.3.3.
6. Alexander Lowen, *The Language of the Body* (New York: Macmillan Publishing Company, 1971), 89.
7. See Alexander Lowen, *Pleasure: A Creative Approach to Life* (New York: Penguin Books, 1975).
8. This understanding of sadism was presented at a small seminar by Dr. Wilhelm Reich, my teacher. I don't believe it was ever published.

CHAPTER 2
1. Masters, William H., and Johnson, Virginia E., *The Human Sexual Response* (Boston: Little, Brown & Co.).

2. L. A. Abramov, "Sexual Life and Sexual Frigidity Among Women Developing Acute Myocardial Infarction," *Psychosomatic Medicine* 38 (December 1976): 418–24.
3. A. J. Wahrer and R. C. Burchell, "Male Sexual Dysfunction Associated with Coronary Heart Disease," *Archives of Sexual Behavior* 9 (1980): 69.
4. Ibid., 70.
5. Wilhelm Reich, *The Function of the Orgasm* (New York: Orgone Institute Press, 1942), 72–87.
6. Lowen, *The Language of the Body*, 81.
7. Reich, op. cit., 79.
8. Marie Robinson, *The Power of Sexual Surrender* (Garden City, N.Y.: Doubleday & Company, 1959).
9. For a full discussion of the Oedipal problem, its cultural origin and its effects on sexuality and personality, see Alexander Lowen, *Fear of Life* (New York: Macmillan Publishing Company, 1980).
10. Alexander Lowen and R. L. Hiewen, *The Way to Vibrant Health* (New York: Harper & Row).

CHAPTER 3

1. This case is fully reported in Alexander Lowen, *Depression and the Body* (New York: Penguin Books, 1972), 166–82.
2. Arthur P. Moyes, *Modern Clinical Psychiatry* (Philadelphia: W. B. Saunders & Company, 1934), 90.
3. Clancy Sigal, "Beware the Forgotten Child in the Marathon Male," *International Herald Tribune*, June 10, 1986.

CHAPTER 4

1. Alexander Lowen, "A Case of Migraine, Bioenergetic Analysis, A Clinical Journal," 1: 117–24.
2. Sigmund Freud, *Mourning and Melancholia*, in *Collected Papers* (London: Hogarth Press, 1953), 4: 152–70.
3. Lowen, *Depression and the Body*, 129–38.

CHAPTER 5

1. For a fuller discussion of the difference between rage and anger, see Alexander Lowen, *Narcissism: Denial of the True Self* (New York: Macmillan Publishing Company, 1983), 93–94.
2. For a full analysis of this personality, see ibid.

CHAPTER 6

1. Meyer Friedman and Diane Ulmer, *Treating Type A Behavior and Your Heart* (New York: Alfred Knopf, 1984), 4.
2. Ibid., 5.
3. Ibid., 144.
4. Stephen Sinatra, unpublished data, based on a ten-year study of admissions for coronary artery disease at Manchester Hospital.
5. I. M. Dombroski et al. Reported by R. B. Williams in *Integrative Psychiatry* 2, no. 4:133.
6. J. C. Barefoal et al. *Psychosomatic Medicine* 45 (1983):13.
7. Friedman and Ulmer, op. cit., 45.
8. Ibid., 31.
9. James Lynch, *The Broken Heart* (New York: Basic Books, 1977).
10. This statistic is age adjusted.
11. Lynch, op. cit., 165.
12. Ibid., 140.
13. Stewart Wolf and Helen Goodell, *Behavioral Science in Clinical Medicine* (Springfield, Ill.: 1926), 79.
14. The mechanism for denial is elaborated in Lowen, *Narcissism*, 56–59.

CHAPTER 7

1. R. Gryglewski, *Prostacycline and Sclerosis* (Wroclaw: Polish Academy of Science, 1981).
2. J. Santorski in ibid., 9.
3. A. M. Master and H. L. Jaffee, "Factors in the Onset of Coronary Occlusion and Coronary Insufficiency: Effort, Occupation, Trauma and Emotion," *JAMA* 148 (1952): 794.
4. C. Avery-Clara, "Sexual Dysfunction and Disorder Patterns of Working and Nonworking Wives," *Journal of Mental Therapy* 12 (1986): 2.
5. Norman Cousins, *The Healing Heart* (New York: W. W. Norton & Company, 1983), 36.
6. Ibid., 35.
7. Barney M. Olin, "Psychobiology and Treatment of Anniversary Reactions," *Psychosomatics* 26 (1986): 505.
8. Ibid., 506.
9. George L. Engel, "Death and Reunion: The Loss of a Twin," *Dartmouth Alumni Magazine*, June 1981.

10. Ibid.
11. Cousins, op. cit., 134.

CHAPTER 8

1. R. A. De Silva and B. Lown, "Ventricular Premature Beats, Stress and Sudden Death," *Psychosomatics* 19 (1978): 694.
2. Ibid., 651.
3. Ibid.
4. Ibid., 650.
5. Ibid.
6. Ibid., 652.
7. A. H. Wellens, A. Venneulen, and D. Duren, "Ventricular Fibrillation Occurring on Arousal from Sleep by Auditory Stimulation," *Circulation* 46 (1972): 661.
8. De Silva and Lown, op. cit., 658.
9. Cousins, *The Healing Heart*, 202.
10. Ibid., 207.
11. Ibid.
12. G. L. Engel, "Sudden and Rapid Death During Psychological Stress," *Annals of Internal Medicine* 74 (1971): 777.
13. M. L. Yawkes, "Emotions as the Cause of Rapid and Sudden Death," *Archives of Neurology and Psychoanalysis* 19 (1936): 875–79; W. B. Cannon, "Voodoo Death," *Psychosomatic Medicine* (1957): 182–90.
14. Cannon, op. cit., 186.
15. J. L. Mathis, "A Sophisticated Version of Voodoo Death, Report of a Case," *Psychosomatic Medicine* 26 (1964): 104–7.

CHAPTER 9

1. Friedman and Ulmer, op. cit., 141.
2. See Lowen, *Fear of Life*, 66–69, for a fuller discussion of this issue.
3. Alexander Lowen, "Some Thoughts About Cancer," *Bioenergetic Analysis* 3, no. 1 (1987): 1–28.

CHAPTER 10

1. Alexander Lowen and Leslie Lowen, *The Way to Vibrant Health: A Manual of Bioenergetic Exercises* (New York: Harper & Row, 1977).

2. Lowen, *Pleasure*, 322.
3. Lowen, *Narcissism*, 324.
4. Erich Fromm, *The Art of Loving* (New York: Harper & Row, 1956), 59.

ARKANA – TIMELESS WISDOM FOR TODAY

With over 150 titles currently in print, Arkana is the leading name in quality books for mind, body, and spirit. Arkana encompasses the spirituality of both East and West, ancient and new. A vast range of interests is covered, including Mythology, Psychology and Transformation, Health, Science and Mysticism, Women's Spirituality, Zen, Western Traditions, and Astrology.

If you would like a catalogue of Arkana books, please write to:

Sales Dept. — Arkana
Penguin USA
375 Hudson St.
New York, NY 10014

Arkana Marketing Department
Penguin Books Ltd.
27 Wrights Lane
London W8 5TZ

DATE DUE

5/24			